GLYCEMIC LOAD CARB COUNTER

GLYCEMIC LOAD CARB COUNTER

✓ GI–GL SMART CHART TABLES™

✓ A–Z FOOD LISTS–ISO AVAILABLE CARBS & GL

✓ YOUR FOODS, YOUR AVAILABLE CARBS, YOUR GL

Judy Lickus BSc, LBSW

JML Publishing

Corpus Christi, TX, USA 78404

Notice

This book is sold with the understanding that the author is not liable for the misconception or misuse of any information provided. The information presented here is in no way intended as a substitute for medical treatment or nutritional counseling.

Links to internet resources are current at time of publication.

Copyright © 2024 by *Judy Lickus, BSc, LBSW*

ISBN: 9798324637866

All rights reserved. No part of this publication may be reproduced or transmitted in any form or by any means, electronic, or mechanical, including photocopying, recording, or any other information storage and retrieval system, without the written permission of the author.

TABLE OF CONTENTS

INTRODUCTION 1

CARBS ARE SPECIAL 3

SUPERCHARGING THE SCIENCE 5

   THE SCIENTIFIC METHOD 5

   ISO EXCEPTIONS 6

      BEER 6

   AVAILABLE CARBS COUNT 7

   ISO STANDARDS AND GLYCEMIC LOAD 8

      PICK YOUR BATTLES 9

      GINGERBREAD 9

      RANGER COOKIES 10

   GI RANKINGS 11

      LOW MEDIUM HIGH GI 11

   THE SCIENCE OF ASSIGNED GI VALUES 13

      THE TREND IS YOUR FRIEND 13

   EMOTIONAL TROUBLESHOOTING 16

      HIGH GI vs LOW GI 17

      ACTIVE vs PASSIVE 18

   DIABETES CARE 19

      TOTAL CARB COUNTS 19

      HYPOGLYCEMIA 20

      GLYCEMIC QUALITY 20

      WORKING WITH YOUR PHYSICIAN 21

      MAINTAINING A LOW GLYCEMIC LOAD 21

   SCIENCE IN THE KITCHEN 23

      COOKING 23

      PPOCESSING 23

      RIPENESS 23

      FIBER 23

COMBINING FOODS...23
CREATING RESISTANT STARCH...24
BREAD 24
FRUITS..24
POTATOES...24
RICE..24
PASTA 24
GRAB & GO SNACK SUGGESTIONS...25

USING SMART CHART TABLES™ 26

BAKERY PRODUCTS ISO 30G AVAIL CARB 34

BEVERAGES ISO 25G AVAIL CARB..37

BREAD & RICE CAKES ISO 15G AVAIL CARB..41

BREAKFAST CEREALS & COOKIES ISO 20G AVAIL CARB................................49

CEREAL GRAINS ISO 45G AVAIL CARB 52

DAIRY & ALTERNATIVES ISO 20G AVAIL CARB..57

FRUIT AND FRUIT PRODUCTS ISO 15G AVAIL CARB...61

LEGUMES ISO 15G AVAIL CARB..69

MEAL REPLACEMENT & WEIGHT MANAGEMENT ISO 20G AVAIL CARB 72

NUTRITIONAL SUPPORT PDTS ISO 30G AVAIL CARB
....77

NUTS ISO 5G AVAIL CARB 79

PASTA ISO 40G AVAIL CARB...80

SNACKS & CONFECTIONERY ISO 25G AVAIL CARB..82

SOUP ISO 20G AVAIL CARB..96

SUGARS & SYRUPS ISO 5G AVAIL CARB 97

VEGETABLES ISO 20G AVAIL CARB...101

TROUBLESHOOTING 108

MEAL PREP NOTES 110

ENDNOTES, REFERENCES & RESOURSES..110

INTRODUCTION

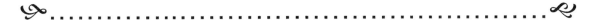

T hank you for taking the time to look inside this book for a peek at the interactive experience that lets you take the reins of your dietary choices. Welcome to *Glycemic Load Carb Counter.*

Glycemic Load Carb Counter is all about carbohydrates. This book looks at Carbs in a special way. This book looks at Carbs through the lens of Glycemic Load. Glycemic Load shows us how a food will affect our blood sugar levels <u>before</u> we eat it. No more waiting for postprandial readings. No more waiting for 3 months, 6 months, or a year for A1C measures to find out how we are doing.

Those glucose readings and A1C numbers are history by the time we get them, and we cannot change history. But the good news is that these are numbers. It's all about the numbers. And the beauty of numbers is that you can always count on them. Numbers are your best friends. This is because Numbers never lie to you. They always tell you the truth.

<u>This is so important, because what you really need to know is</u> how the foods you regularly eat affect you. And we are going to use numbers to get to the bottom of this. Discover the foods that spike your blood sugar and those that keep it mellow. You deserve to know. Now there will be more falling for Tony the Tiger sugarcoating everything. The cat is now out of the bag, so to speak, and you are finally in charge!

Glycemic Load Carb Counter comes complete with tables of the Glycemic Index (GI) and Glycemic Load (GL) of many foods. To top it all off, you will have up-to-date scientific GI and GL test results that you may need going forward including beer, tomato juice, and even human breast milk. And you can use this information to inform your choices before you get to the cash register.

But that's not all. This interactive book brings you so much more than just the GI Rankings and GL Scores of specific foods. This book gives you a whole lot more than that. In this book, you can keep track of your own serving sizes as you chart your course to low glycemic load eating, one personalized serving at a time.

By the way, links to all of the resources used in the creation of this book are included in the Endnotes, References & Resources section at the end of the book for your convenience.

'Glycemic Load Carb Counter' is more than just a book. With this dynamic new tool, you can tailor nutritional insights to meet your own unique needs.

You will come to appreciate the power of Glycemic Index and Glycemic Load in a way you never have before. It may even save your life.

Are you ready to chart your course to balanced eating, one personalized serving at a time? Whether you are a Blood Sugar Balancer, Weight Loss Manager, Diabetes Diet Designer or just a healthy eater, the best tool does the best job.

This dynamic new tool puts you right on the cutting edge of your own healthcare.

Because with Glycemic Load Carb Counter, you are not just a reader. You are the captain on your own journey to improved health and vitality.

So, why settle for less when there is more to be had?

CARBS ARE SPECIAL

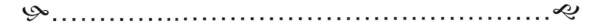

When we talk about the food we eat, we focus on three main types of food: proteins, fats, and carbohydrates. These three main types of foods are *macro*nutrients, and make up most of the foods we eat. These three foods make up the bulk of our diets.

This illustration below funnels these three main types of foods to point out the type of macronutrient we are looking at in this book with a checkmark. ✓

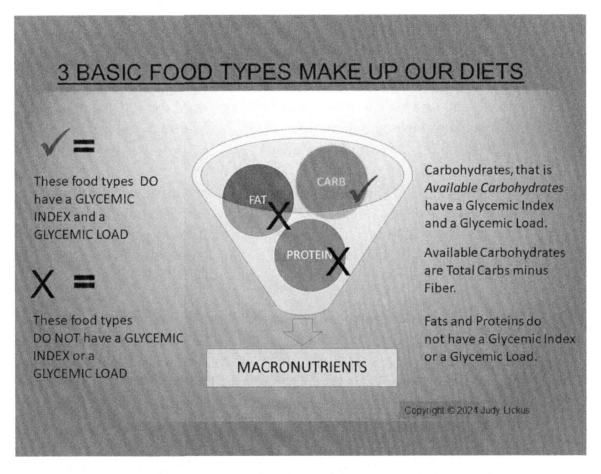

Fat and Protein do not raise our blood sugar levels. Carbohydrates are special foods because they do affect our blood sugar levels. And we use Glycemic Index (GI) to show us how much each different type of Carbohydrate can affect our blood sugar. It's a way to "grade" the carbs in our lives. We can use Glycemic Index GI when picking out our food.

Now, when we talk about the Glycemic Index, we only look at a certain kind of carbs called "Available Carbs." That is because with Glycemic Index, only Available Carbs Count! These are the kind of carbs our bodies easily digest. This way, we narrow down our focus to the important "impactful" part of the Carbs. To get the Available Carbs in a food, we subtract the Fiber from the Total Carbs.

And do you know what else? Authentic Glycemic Index tables include only foods that have Available Carbs because those are the Carbs that have real impact on our blood sugar levels. And as a matter of fact, only Available Carbs count when we use the power of Glycemic Load to make our dreams come true.

Why waste our time or space with foods that have no Carbohydrate, right? All we need to understand is what really matters most when it comes to the food we eat. And what matters most is the power of some Carbs to affect our blood sugar more than others. Now our job is to ferret these out and fix things up to keep our blood glucose mellow.

It's not like we have to invent the wheel. Researchers have made great strides in Blood Glucose management for over the past one hundred years. Countless lives have been lost to long-term high blood glucose levels, and many lives are still being lost today. Why should any of us lose when we can all win?

We have come a long way since Frederick Banting's team discovered that insulin from dogs works in humans, too. The latest trend is the use of injectable GLP-1 drugs. But wait a minute, isn't that the hormone they use to bring livestock to market faster? These drugs fool our bodies, cost thousands of dollars a year, and deliver some major side effects. Maybe if we had no other choice, we might be thankful.

However, there is a far better way. And all it takes is a bit of our time and the simple arithmetic we learned in fifth grade.

And there are even some things we can do to expand on our success. As you read on, you will discover some clever ways to supercharge the science and fine-tune your results.

Let's get to it!

SUPERCHARGING THE SCIENCE

This book would not be complete if we overlooked some of the science of why our success is possible. And it's best we start off with just that goal in mind. What some may consider nit picking, others may think of as fine-tuning. No matter how you look at it, there are some details that we can use to our advantage. These are the kind of details we can use to "supercharge" the results we get from the science.

So to begin with, we need to understand science. We need to realize the nature of science to make the best use of it in our lives.

THE SCIENTIFIC METHOD
When we are working with science, we must be exact. We want our details to be precise because Science holds itself to what is called the "Scientific Method." Now according to the Scientific Method, Scientists start out with a "hypothesis," for their study. It might be some theory or assumption that they have. Alternatively, It may be an idea they want to investigate that they think is the cause of something. Then they create a plan for a study or design a research project that puts their idea to the test.

The Scientific Method requires that study <u>results</u> MUST reproduce themselves when using the same inputs. Kind of like "cause and effect." AND it has to happen repeatedly. Kind of like doing the same thing over and over and getting the same result. This is how they prove the validity of their idea. We will call upon the scientific method again as we go through the upcoming topics.

In this chapter, we are all about digging into the science. Some of the topics we will cover include:

- ISO Exceptions to Avail Carbs
- Available Carbs Count
- ISO Standards and Glycemic Load
- GI Rankings
- The Science of Assigned GI Values
- Emotional Troubleshooting
- Diabetes Care
- Science in the Kitchen
- Using Smart Chart Tables™

ISO EXCEPTIONS

In this book, foods are in Sixteen ISO Food Categories. Three of these categories have exceptions to the number of ISO Assigned Avail Carbs used to calculate GL per serving. The categories are "Beverages," "Dairy & Alternatives", and "Vegetables." Exceptions are marked with an asterisk (*) for your convenience.

So, for example, let's take a closer look at the Beverage Category. The Beverage Category has ISO Assigned Available Carbs of 25 g, (as you can see in the header of the chapter titled Beverages). Now, the first big issue to keep in mind with beverages is that our bodies digest them so fast. There is no chewing to slow things down. So beverages act like liquid glucose.

However, there are exceptions to using 25 g Avail Carbs for some beverages. For instance, beer, human breast milk, and tomato juice are exceptions in the Beverage Category. For these, ISO recommends only 10g Available Carbs to calculate Glycemic Load. Any exceptions like this are marked with an asterisk so you do not miss them.

BEER
We'll take a closer look at beer, which may have about 12 g of Carbs in a can. How does a beer shake out in terms GI? The three tested beers all have a High GI. They come in at 119, 89, and 80. Beer has an ISO Assigned Avail Carb of only 10 rather than 25 to calculate GL. Tested beers deliver a GL of 12, another 9, and a non-alcoholic version comes in at 8. Keep in mind that these results are based on 10 g Avail Carb per serving.

However, if we calculated beer for GL using 25 g of Avail Carbs, like other beverages, Beer would have a GL that could be as high as 30 per serving. Ouch. Talk about being over-served at the pub!

Now, if you can locate a very low carb beer, let's say 5 g Avail Carb per serving, even if it has a GI as high as 119, that beer would have a GL of only 6. But do check your blood glucose levels here, as some report that even half a very low carb beer can cause a spike.

Your best bet on an unknown and unstudied beer is to sip on it for an hour.

Next, we will take a closer look at getting those important accurate Available Carb Counts.

AVAILABLE CARBS COUNT

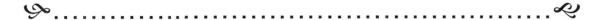

As you could see in the example of Beer we just looked at, those Available Carbs are important. In many cases, getting accurate counts may not be as simple as we expect. You may need to do a bit of additional research. A few options meet the test of the Scientific Method. The United States Department of Agriculture (USDA) and the Food and Drug Association have standardized our food labeling practices. So, one option as a potential consumer is to read the "Nutrition Fact" label on prepared foods. These labels must include the Total Carb grams and Fiber grams per serving. Total Carb grams minus Fiber grams give you the Avail Carb grams you need to calculate Your GL.

A second option might be to enter "Available carbohydrate in 'name of the food' + USDA" in your search bar. At least this gets you the first result from the USDA, Food Data Central. General "searches" for online results are unreliable. Many offer conflicting, and frequently incorrect information. So this why I recommend the third option.

In the case of less complex foods and foods that don't have a Nutrition Fact label, you'll likely head over to this next option.

The third option is the one I most highly recommend. This is an exceptional online resource. I like to use this for times when I will be looking up some carb counts. So here's an idea. When you are on your computer, head over to the USDA National Nutrient Database at Food Data Central.[1] You can "pin" this website to your toolbar to keep it handy as you do your food research.

At Food Data Central (aka FDC), you can search for brand specific prepared foods, plain natural foods, and just plain ingredients to get the amount of Available Carbs in any food. FDC reports "Carbohydrate by Difference." Carbohydrate by difference means the remaining Available Carbs after removing everything else from the food.

All of this underscores the importance of Available Carbs. Because when it comes to Carbs and our blood sugar levels, only Available Carbs count.

Now we will turn our attention to ISO Standards and see how they help us arrive at a Low Glycemic Load.

---

[1] https://fdc.nal.usda.gov/

ISO STANDARDS AND GLYCEMIC LOAD

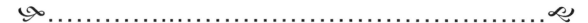

The older International Tables measured by serving size, in weight or volume. They reported Available Carbs based on the serving size. The new International Tables measure by Available Carbs rather than serving size. The new ISO Standards on calculating Glycemic Load use the same amount of Available Carbs for each food within their food group. These new Tables are truly standardized. When we use the same amount of Available Carbs for each of the foods, we can quickly see how one food really compares to another, carb to carb, so to speak.

This standardizes the measuring of the purest part of the food that effects blood glucose levels. When you measure all the foods the same way, you can see how they really compare to one another based on what matters most. Not only that, because you measure them all the same way, you are truly in line with the Scientific Method. We will talk more about the Scientific Method soon.

Using the new International Tables may seem confusing if you are used to using the older International Tables. So it may take a bit of time to get the hang of using them. But compared to older International Tables, the new ISO standards can be much more useful to us as we design the Glycemic Load (GL) of our servings. Let me count some ways.

As we look at the Smart Chart Table of Bakery Products, for example, we can get a much faster idea about the GL of the different choices we can make.

Now we can finally see at-a-glance comparisons of the Glycemic Load (GL) of different choices based on the GI and the amount of Available Carb consumed. And all it takes is a glance.

In contrast to the older tables, this new way of measuring says nothing about the actual volume or even the weight of food in a serving. But we need an answer to an important question. How much can you eat of each one and still be in line with your Low Glycemic Load lifestyle?

To answer this burning question, we will look at the evidence. Bakery Products are foods that are typically high in carbs. And none of the entries from the new International Tables qualify as a low Glycemic Load serving. Not one. But this is where it gets interesting. There is no rule that says we have to eat a 30 g carb portion of any bakery product. So the 30 g Available Carb used for calculating Glycemic Load (GL) is our useful information.

What can we do with this information? Creating a trend for a group of foods gives us a crystal clear comparison of the glycemic potential of each food. This way we might consider another selection within the group. So, as we look over the other foods in the group, we can instantly spot the closest low Glycemic Load options. Maybe we want to try something else instead of what we had in mind.

PICK YOUR BATTLES

It gets really personal here, because each of us have our own preferences. There is always more than one choice. And we do have the freedom to choose from many choices. But in the end, it always comes down to one choice or another. So we have to pick our battles. Now what can we do if we REALLY want to have our cake and eat it, too?

And what if that cake happens to be Starbucks Gingerbread Loaf? OK, then. Let's take a closer look at that. One serving is 118 g. So that's like 4 ounces. It delivers 63 g Available Carbs. And we're looking at a HIGH GI of 89. Hmmm. Sounds pretty serious. And you've been grabbing one of these each day for your afternoon snack with your coffee? I see. Yes, this is serious.

GINGERBREAD

Consider this: Gingerbread Cake has the highest GL of all Bakery Products. Most Bakery Products have a GL between 12 and 27. Let's say you still have your heart set on Gingerbread Cake, weighing in with a GL of 27. Is there any way you want to pick something else instead? No? Is that your answer, no? OK. Then here is your best move.

You help yourself to a serving size that contains only 10 g Available Carbs. So that is about 1/3 of the slice. Total size of slice is 118 g. Divide by 3, that's 39 g. weight or one and a half ounces in total. Maybe two small bites. That Gingerbread Cake sure must be delicious, so you can savor each bite and enjoy it while it just melts in your mouth. Now you put the rest away for the next two days, and save yourself some health and money. Don't like this answer? I didn't like it either. Ok, we'll look at some options.

So I figured maybe an updated Gingerbread recipe could fulfill my craving. But I couldn't find any that met my need for low Glycemic Load. In order to get my way, I had to invent my own recipe. Gingerbread Baby-Cakes. I figured a recipe for 12 cupcakes would be the way to go. That way I'd get 12 servings. And I knew that the HIGH GI Wheat-flour in the Starbucks Loaf was raising both the GI and the Available Carbs. So I knew where to start.

Comparing Gingerbread Options

Nutrition	Starbucks® Gingerbread Loaf	Gingerbread Baby-Cakes
Available Carbs	64	16
GI	89	55
GL	27	9
Calories	380	81
Fiber	1	2

Here's how the numbers looked. For a GI of 89 at Starbucks, mine had a GI of 55. For the 64 g Available Carbs at Starbucks, mine had only 16. This meant that mine had less than a third of theirs, another bonus. But the most important fact it all boiled down to is this: My GL is only 9 compared to their GL of 27.

For me, this option worked out really well. The numbers looked fine, and I had a safe fix for my sweet tooth. And all it took was an hour on a Saturday afternoon and I had 12 of them. I even got to eat an entire cupcake in the end! This way I could freeze the rest, and grab one on my way out the door in the morning as I wish. Goes great with a piece of fresh fruit or a small bowl of berries.

RANGER COOKIES

I included some alternative ingredients and a couple recipes from my book "Are You Sweet Enough Already" in the Smart Chart Tables™ in this book to give you some ideas to work with. The dessert recipes have nutrition information including GI and GL for each serving. All have a Glycemic Load of 10 or less. *Look Inside* that book at Amazon and grab the Ranger Cookie recipe free. And you can eat six of those for a serving! And you still have a low Glycemic Load! You don't have to buy the book. This is just to give you some recipe ideas. The Ranger Cookie recipe is my gift to you. I want to celebrate with you as you take the next step to help yourself.

I know that at first it can seem hard to figure a Low Glycemic Load. But in the end, it is so worth it. Sure it takes a bit of our time and some thoughtful planning at first. Getting creative in the kitchen is a long-term investment that will pay you great health dividends over time. Now we'll turn our attention to general "GI Rankings" of our Available Carbs.

GI RANKINGS

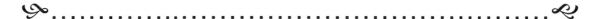

A very popular way to look at Glycemic Index (GI) is to use the Low, Medium, High approach. In this approach, GI Rankings fall into three general categories as shown in this little table below:

Glycemic Index Rankings:

| Low GI = 0-55 |
| Medium GI = 56-69 |
| High GI = 70+ |

LOW MEDIUM HIGH GI

Notice how all these rankings have a "range." This way of looking at GI Rankings might be a good first step for beginning beginners. You can target 55 or less for Low GI. That is a great start. But over the long term, you will want the actual scientific results as tested on human test subjects so you can maintain a Low Glycemic Load. This is how you will really make a difference in your blood glucose levels. You need this for the long term. Why bother with all this researching and arithmetic unless you are going to use the right numbers? What's the point?

Consider how "Low GI" goes up to 55. That is a 55-point range, right? And at 55 you are only one point away from Medium GI. So how can you calculate GL? When you figure GL, you really need the actual GI of the specific Carb, not just a range. Sure, it may be tricky getting the hang of it right away. However, doing the job right gets you the right results. Anything short of that and you are accepting a very broad estimate over an actual number. How can you measure the fact? Wait a minute you won't even have a fact, you will have a range.

That is the important thing about Glycemic Load. And you need to calculate it to have it. I like to say that when you have the real GI Ranking and Avail Carbs, the GL falls right into your hands. But it starts with the right numbers. How you are going to do some 5th grade arithmetic with only an estimate? How will you get a result you can count on unless you use the correct numbers?

It's really about the science of blood sugar. Ranges are fine if you are only interested in understanding a general idea. But ranges fall far short when you understand the idea and want to apply the underlying science to get real life results. If you really want to work with the science, you want to work with the exact numbers.

Much, but not all of this holds true for "Assigned GI Rankings" as well, and we will talk about Assigned GI Rankings in a minute. And it is true as we just discussed, we will not know the GI of a food exactly until we have a GI test result. And while Assigned GI is a much more evolved idea and it is only an idea about a particular food (not truly certain until testing), it does give us something much closer than a range to work with. That's the reason it brings us so much closer to the truth of a food than the LOW, MEDIUM, or HIGH Range idea ever could! So next we are going to look at the Science of Assigned GI Rankings.

In the meantime, to grab a hold of the pure science and use the real numbers is where you will have great success.

GLYCEMIC LOAD CARB COUNTER

THE SCIENCE OF ASSIGNED GI VALUES

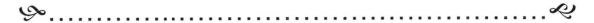

There are times when even our best efforts do not bring us the answers we seek. These are times when we may feel limited in what we can do. But we know how important it is to do the best we can. It's like we can't do everything, but we can do some things. And what we can do, we must do. Then what we must do, we shall do. Because it is just that important.

At times like these, we work with the best we can get.

THE TREND IS YOUR FRIEND
It is at times like these, that the trend is your friend. And in this case, the trend is the power of Assigned GI Rankings. Now we'll take a closer look at how we've established this trend.

To date, scientists have tested and published the results of GI Rankings and GL Scores for nearly 5,000 foods from all over the world. While this may sound like a lot, and it is, according to National Geographic's January 2024 issue, there are over 50,000 different edible plants on our earth! Our blessings are so abundant that we may, in fact, never have full results of GI testing for all of these edible plants! And this is even before they have become "ingredients" in our many recipes! So how will we know we have the right numbers to do our arithmetic with?

We will go directly to the most reliable source of all for our scientific data. The data we want has been put to the test of the "Scientific Method" that we talked about earlier.

The National Institutes of Health, commonly referred to as NIH or PubMed, is the primary agency of the US Government responsible for Biomedical and Public Health research. NIH houses the National Library of Medicine. This is the largest biomedical library in the world. NIH is the national resource for health professionals, scientists, as well as the public. I go to NIH when I am serious for deep learning about a subject. By this, I mean I want to read the exact science of it. I want to have my own ideas after reading about a discovery. And I know that these are rigorously peer-reviewed articles published through the NIH. And they bring us to the solid core of the science we need to make our own best decisions.

Now here comes that trend that is our friend again. The simple table below shows the Assigned GI Values for some foods that may not be listed or even specifically tested for their GI. But first, let's look at how this trend came about.

In 1981, David Jenkins introduced the idea of a Glycemic Index (GI). GI is a scale that goes from one to one hundred. It lets us compare how rapidly different Available Carbs break down during digestion. Scientists already knew that protein foods like eggs, meat, poultry, and wild game did not raise blood glucose levels. They knew the same was true for fats and oils, as well. So protein foods do not have a GI, nor do fats and oils.

Over the years, after testing hundreds of dairy products, scientists learned that natural, unsweetened dairy products have an average GI of 30. Fruits and vegetables, on the other hand average out to a GI of 40. (One rainy day I even did the math on all the fruits to be certain.) And wheat flour products, those weigh in with an average GI of 70. Seems clear-cut, right?

It becomes complex as we add flour to meat to make gravy. Adding flour adds GI factors. We are no longer eating just the meat. The addition of flour, of course, creates a GI of 70 in the gravy, whereas the addition of fat to the mix will lower the GL.

So for now, this table might come in handy when you are looking for a GI on a specific food not listed in NIH published international tables. This way at least you can play the trend as they did with the dairy, fruits and veggies, and wheat flour products.

And with over 40,000 foods to go, the trend may be our best friend for a good long while. The table also includes a few basic "GI" free foods like protein and fats just as a reminder. This is kind of like a "Rule of Thumb" idea. Something to keep in mind to save your time as you learn the GI of specific foods. Also helpful as you shop, just to have a good idea of what you might be adding to your cart when you are just beginning.

Keep in mind that this little table is for plain, natural foods. Animal protein foods like meat, fish, poultry, and eggs do not have carbohydrate. Plain fats and oils do not have carbohydrates either. Therefore, these foods do not have a glycemic index. For the sake of saving space and your valuable time, this book is for working with foods that contain carbohydrate.

Assigned and Natural GI Values for Unlisted Products

Food Type	GI
Animal protein like Eggs, Meat, Poultry, Wild game, plain	0
Fats and oils, plain	0
Dairy Products, plain	30
Fruits & Vegetables	40
Wheat Flour Products	70

As you can see, it is a pretty brief table. But goes straight to the point and sums up what we are working with. Remember the three food types we talked about in the beginning of the book: Protein, fat, and carbohydrate? And we said that carbohydrates are the only food type with a GI. This little table tells you to use a GI of 30 for unlisted dairy, for fruits and veggies use 40, and for wheat flour products use 70 for GI. Dairy, fruits and veggies, and wheat flour all contain Carbs. Now that might save you hundreds of pages of research!

Now we are going to take a look at how our emotions can help us recognize when we can benefit from using GL and GL to make our dreams come true.

EMOTIONAL TROUBLESHOOTING

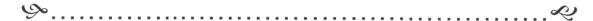

There is a powerful warning sign we need to talk about. This warning sign is a good signal telling us when we might have more moving around to do. It could also tell us that we are working with the wrong numbers. Now we are talking about our emotions.

In the following diagram, a black arrow highlights an important timeframe in the eating of HIGH GI foods. The time is about an hour and a half after eating the HIGH GI food. This is when Blood Glucose levels to fall to a level that is lower than they were before eating.

And this continues for the next few hours as blood glucose continues to fall.

(I know I covered this subject thoroughly with loads of data and links to research for you in *Glycemic Load Food Guide.* However, I do not want my new readers to miss out on this powerful bit of insight.)

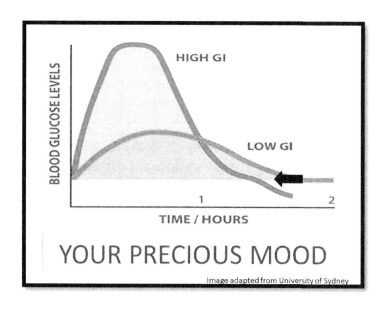

If you happen to be dealing with feelings of sadness, tiredness, or depression, in your life, and you can't figure out the reason, it may be due to the foods you are eating. How can you tell? You might like to take the time to notice your emotions starting at the timeframe of the arrow point in the above diagram. This marks the time when you might begin to notice unpleasant symptoms. It's also when your blood sugar falls below where it was before you ate.

HIGH GI vs LOW GI

As you may expect, in just the first few minutes after eating a HIGH GI food, your energy level skyrockets, and it might even feel like you have a super power. You might even feel like you could shingle a barn. These excited, euphoric feelings can continue for about as long as the dark red line stays higher than it was before you last ate. So right off the bat, you have extra energy.

Maybe 20 minutes later, you'll start to slide down. But just before that, you may notice that you feel at a plateau for maybe 15 minutes or so. Your feelings settle down to a comfortable level. But soon your body runs out of that "happy juice." Your body dispatches all the extra glucose. It might take half an hour to an hour, but it is heading back down. And you can feel it. And it's going down to a level below where it was at before you ate the HIGH GI food.

So, starting about an hour after eating a HIGH GI food, take a few deep, centering breaths. Collect your thoughts, put them aside, and focus on your body. Notice how you are feeling. Check in with yourself to see if you, too, are experiencing a dramatic spike and dramatic crash of blood glucose levels around these times. For many of us, the emotional consequences are great indeed. This is especially true of foods we eat regularly. And it is exceptionally true if we eat certain HIGH GI foods daily. At this point, bless this as the warning sign that it is.

There is so much more that we can gain when we pay attention to the impact of the foods we eat on our emotional selves.

You might find it helpful to keep a journal on this impact of eating High GI foods. Take note of the day, time, specific food, Serving Size, Available Carbs, and the Glycemic Load of your serving. There is a Troubleshooter for you following the Smart Chart Tables™ where you can add your own inputs to keep track of things like this.

And don't overlook the matter of personal response to foods. Where one food may spike blood glucose for one person, a second person may not have as strong a reaction. It will be helpful to you to keep track of your own responses.

You see, on a very personal level, when we eat HIGH GI foods, our Blood Glucose level spikes. This spike summons our pancreatic islets of Langerhans into action. Our islets of Langerhans pump out, to the best of their ability, enough insulin to manage the spike back down to a healthy level. Thank goodness for that. But the whole process creates a lot of short-term extra energy just to move the extra glucose around.

ACTIVE vs PASSIVE

What happens to all the extra energy created during this process? That depends on how we decide to deal with the extra energy. The question is are we active or are we passive?

When we are active, we raise our metabolism to burn it off. Getting moving in any fashion will do the trick. Even just walking around for fifteen or twenty minutes after a meal will help take care of the spike and burn off the energy. How miraculous our body is!

However, if we are passive, and just sit around after our meals, our body cannot burn it off. Instead, the insulin created to soothe the spike in our Blood Glucose caused by eating HIGH GI Carbs … directs all of that extra energy right into our fat cells. That's right, the insulin drives it right into our fat cells for storage in time of need. And when you think about it, isn't this the job of insulin?

While this may have come in handy during times of famine in the era of our hunting/gathering days, it may no longer suit us in our lives today. But it worked perfectly for us a hundred years ago when we had to catch our fish on a tree branch.

So now, we know what is ours to choose to do.

Nowhere is all of this more important than for those dealing a with type 2 diabetes.

DIABETES CARE

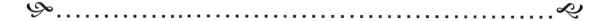

Physicians do get one class (for one semester) on nutrition in medical school. But the only way they learn about Glycemic Index is to do their own research in their own spare time.

So far, nutrition care is not part of the managed health care systems we have in place today. It is as if our nutrition had nothing to do with us.

And it takes a humble and honest physician to own up to the fact that the best they have to offer are drugs for our symptoms.

They learn about emergency care, thank goodness. They learn about medicine. They learn about health, and what it looks like. They learn about disease, and what that looks like. And we appreciate all of that a lot.

So when it comes to a diabetes diagnosis, they know the numbers to look for. They know all the symptoms. They know about the complications that develop due to inefficient diabetes control. They also know that yes, it can kill you. And when you deal with neuropathy, kidney disease, and loss of vision, there are other waiting rooms you have to wait in to see even more doctors for more symptoms. And yet, they all address the symptoms but not the underlying cause.

And this is what the physician learned in medical school. He learned how to prescribe medicine to help relieve the discomfort caused by these additional symptoms. So he can now help tend to the complications. Many of which are caused by our inefficient system of diabetes control. But unfortunately, during his education, the physician hardly even considered how our nutrition can affect our health.

I just think that as a society we can do a whole lot better job managing this. Putting the Glycemic Index (GI) and Glycemic Load (GL) on every manufactured food product label would be a nice start. And including this information on our National Nutrient Databases would be great.

TOTAL CARB COUNTS
So if you have a diagnosis of type 2 Diabetes, it is off to a Diabetes Educator you go. These Diabetes Educators work for the American Diabetes Association. And they teach you how to dose yourself with external insulin. They teach you to dose based on the Total Carbs in a meal. The next few paragraphs address this most popular method.

First, for many of us this may be a good start. We have to start somewhere! And at least there is some help available. But this approach is missing some of the most important information that we could use to control our blood sugar ourselves. And we'll get into that shortly, but first we need to talk about the consequences of giving our body too much insulin.

HYPOGLYCEMIA
When we dose our insulin based only on Total Carb counts, we can find ourselves with hypoglycemia (low blood sugar). This is when our blood sugar level falls below 70 mg/dl. It is nothing to fool around with. And it can even cause a loss of consciousness.

If or when this happens, the usual advice is to eat glucose tablets to raise your blood sugar back up to a healthy level. So you need to keep these glucose tablets handy in case, or for when this happens to you.

So, now let's look at why our dosing external insulin based on those Total Carb counts can put you in this situation.

In the first place, Total Carbs include:

- Insoluble (indigestible) fiber,
- Some sugar alcohols (like erythritol), and
- Resistant starches that do not raise our blood sugar levels.

The above Carbs are all included in "Total Carb" counts. And we raise the amount of insulin we inject in order to manage them. While in reality, the Carbs listed above do not raise our blood glucose levels. If anything, some can lower our blood sugar levels. Can you see why dosing insulin based on Total Carbs can easily cause an error of overestimation?

As if that is not bad enough, another reason hypoglycemia may occur is because Total Carb counts have no respect for the *glycemic quality* (GI) of a food. That's right; Total Carbs do not care about the fact that some Carbs raise our blood sugar higher than others do.

GLYCEMIC QUALITY
One Carb may burn like a gentle flame, whereas another may burn like a roaring bonfire. Total Carb counts do not care one bit about this important difference. But the Glycemic Load tells you all that before you even eat the food. Do you see the error in the thinking here? It matters. This is another reason why dosing our external insulin based only on Total Carbs can cause us to overshoot our goal and end up with hypoglycemia.

It can even happen when we combine protein and/or fat with the Carbs in a meal. This is because protein and fat slow down the digestion and absorption of food. So when dosing based on Total Carbs only, too much insulin may be present before the carbs are even digested, causing hypoglycemia.

Physical activity is good for us. But it raises our metabolism, which lowers the level of glucose in our blood. So this is also something else we need to keep in mind when dosing external insulin based on our Total Carb counts. And of course, this, too can cause hypoglycemia.

As you can see, there are so many reasons why we want to do better than just counting Total Carbs. Maybe it's time to take the matter into our own hands.

When we use Glycemic Load (GL), we can learn so much about a food before we eat it. Glycemic Load shows us how high a food can make our blood sugar go. This way we can avoid the surprise of skyrocketing blood sugar … or the perils of hypoglycemia.

WORKING WITH YOUR PHYSICIAN

Working with a trusted physician is important. Always consult with your physician when making decisions about your care. The answer may lie in temporary use of a Continuous Glucose Monitor (CGM) of some sort until you get things under control.

For someone who wishes to maintain a low glycemic load lifestyle, that equates to about a daily glycemic load of 50. So, this is like five meals a day (including snacks) that each have a GL of 10 or less.

If your calculation shows a GL that is more than 10 (the limit for a low Glycemic Load), you can reduce your serving size. This lowers the amount of Available Carb, and effectively reduces the GL.

Alternative sweeteners, such as Stevia, with a GI of "0," will reduce the GI in any recipes as compared to other sugar, honey, or syrup. This lowers the GL as well. Other sweeteners are included in the Smart Chart Tables™ in the section "Sugars & Syrups."

MAINTAINING A LOW GLYCEMIC LOAD

Maintaining a daily low GL limit of 50 GL has proven to lead to life changing results in many clients with T2D. Many who had gone beyond metformin to insulin injections turned their lives around by using GL. But it does take some time. And a bit of thought and planning. But the fact is that they found they could reduce and stop these treatments as their blood sugar levels normalized by maintaining their Low GL diet over several months.

Maintaining a low Glycemic Load is very powerful. Please keep in mind that since you no longer spike your blood sugar levels as you did in the past, you will need less external insulin. Consult with your physician to determine the right amount of insulin for you.

If you are on diabetic medications, it is important to test your blood sugar levels frequently. This is especially important as you begin to see and feel the good results as you work with Glycemic Load (GL).

Experienced clients report feeling full all the time, while some are thrilled at losing 50 pounds in 6 months. Don't be fooled by the simplicity. Results can be dramatic when we use the science.

Next, we will explore some tips and techniques we have learned from science that help us prepare and serve our meals with a lower GI and GL.

SCIENCE IN THE KITCHEN

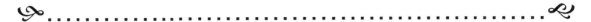

In this section, we consider various ways we can reduce GI and in turn GL of some of our favorite foods.

COOKING
Boiling, microwaving, or steaming usually keeps the GI of foods lower than baking or frying.

Foods cooked for a long time or at high temperatures usually have a higher GI.

PPOCESSING
Processed foods like white bread or white rice have such a high GI because much of their nutrients and fiber are removed during processing.

Whole grain foods, including whole wheat bread and brown rice, have a lower GI because they contain more fiber. Check your Ingredients and the Nutrition Facts labels. Whole grain breads list whole grain as the first ingredient.

RIPENESS
Ripe fruits, like bananas, have a higher GI because their starches turn into sugars as they ripen.

So fruits that are less ripe usually have a lower GI.

FIBER
Foods that are high in fiber tend to have a lower GI and GL. Fiber helps slow down the digestion process and can prevent blood sugar levels from rising too quickly.

Beginning our meals with high fiber foods, like a salad or vegetables slows down the digestion of the entire meal.

COMBINING FOODS
The way we combine different foods can affect the overall GI and GL of our meals.

Including foods like vegetables, whole grains, and legumes in your diet lowers the GI and GL of the entire meal.

Including protein, healthy fats, or foods with low GI in a meal lower the overall GL of the meal. For example, having fish, poultry or avocado with a meal that includes high GI foods lowers the GL and helps balance the blood sugar response.

Including protein or healthy fats in a meal with high GI foods, like rice or bread, can help lower the GI and GL of the meal.

CREATING RESISTANT STARCH
1. For any starchy food, like potatoes, rice, and pasta, cooking and cooling before eating lowers the GI.
2. For any starchy food, cooking, cooling, and refrigerating overnight lowers the GI further.
3. For any starchy food, cooking, cooling, refrigerating overnight and reheating before eating lowers the GI even further yet.
4. The above treatments increase the "Resistant Starch" in starchy foods. But none of these treatments reduces the Available Carb Counts.

BREAD
Whole grain bread has a lower GI than white bread because it contains more fiber. But check the Ingredients label to be sure it is whole grain.

FRUITS
Unripe fruits contain a lot of resistant starch. Ripe fruits like bananas have a higher GI than unripe ones because the starches break down into sugars as they ripen.

Eating fat or protein with a meal lowers the GL of fruits because fat and protein slow down digestion.

POTATOES
Mashed potatoes have a lower GI than baked, because they usually contain butter or milk.

Eating potatoes with the skin on lowers the GI because the skin has fiber that slows down digestion.

Red potatoes, sweet potatoes and yams have a lower GI than white potatoes.

RICE
Brown rice still has its outer layer (or bran, a fiber) intact. White rice has a high GI because processing removes the outer layer (or bran, a fiber) from White rice.

When you cook starches like rice, let it cool down before eating. This can lower the GI because cooling changes the structure of the starch.

PASTA
Cooking pasta al dente (firm to the bite) creates a lower GI than when you cook it longer. The softer your pasta becomes, the more it is already broken down before you eat it, leaving little work for digestion.

By being aware of these facts, we can make smart choices in the ways we cook, combine, and serve our foods. This way we can help keep blood sugar levels steady and maintain a healthy diet.

And last but not least, here is a little list of some foods you might like to keep on hand. These foods all have very few Carbs and a very low GI.

GRAB & GO SNACK SUGGESTIONS

> **Some Foods with Little-to-No Carbs/Glycemic Index Make Great Snacking Food Ideas:**
>
> | | |
> |---|---|
> | Hard boiled egg | Shrimp |
> | Dill pickle | Swiss Chard, Red or Green |
> | Celery stalks | Lettuce, any kind |
> | Broccoli | Yellow Squash |
> | Romaine lettuce – roll-up> | Cold cuts (meat, poultry) |
> | Raw Carrots | Zucchini Squash |
> | Hummus (chickpea dip) | Olives |
> | Baby Spring Mix | Sunflower, pumpkin seeds |
> | Cheeses | Radish |
> | Avocado | Spinach |
> | Nuts, Peanuts, Pistachios | Nopalito |

Keeping a supply of some of your favorites from the above list ready to go can come in handy. Already sliced and eager to serve, enjoy them any time you like. These are just a few ideas; you will likely discover more of them as you review the Smart Chart Tables™. A nice assortment makes great Road Fuel for your travels. Armed with healthy foods, it is easy to avoid unhealthy temptations as you enjoy your new lifestyle. A major benefit of keeping a Low Glycemic Load Lifestyle is that you never need to be hungry!

Now we turn our attention to using the Smart Chart Tables™. The following section details the step-by-step process for you.

USING SMART CHART TABLES™

The tables of this book have three sets of columns, with three columns in each set.

Here is how we use these nine columns to make our dreams come true:

❖ **First three columns** present reference information regarding specific foods:

1. <u>PubRef#</u>: Shows you the science study and the number of each foods' test result.

2. <u>ISO Assigned Category</u>: Wondering what's up with "ISO Assigned Category"? ISO stands for *The International Standards Organization*. ISO is a group that decides the best way to group and measure different types of food. This helps us know what nutrients and benefits we get from each group of food. In this way, the ISO helps make it easier for us to choose the right kinds of food. We use sixteen ISO categories to group the foods in this book. A few foods, like corn, fruit, and vegetable juices appear in more than one category for your convenience.

3. <u>Food & Food Details</u>: Shows the names of foods, and may include prep and serving tips that reduce the Glycemic Index (GI).

❖ **Second three columns** have a greyed background. These numbers stay the same and show up here for your reference. These are the results of scientific testing of individual foods on human test subjects. This is what you use to figure out the Glycemic Load (GL) of your own servings.

4. <u>GI</u>: The GI column shows you the Glycemic Index (GI) Rank of each carbohydrate food. GI is the scientific measure of how high and how fast a carbohydrate food can raise blood sugar when we eat it. GI Rank lets us compare the glycemic essence of different foods per gram of carbohydrate. In other words, this is the personality of the food. You will use this GI Rank number as you calculate Your GL in the third set of columns.

The following image is a reminder to of the effects of HIGH GI foods (shown in dark red) and LOW GI foods (shown in light yellow) on blood glucose levels after eating.

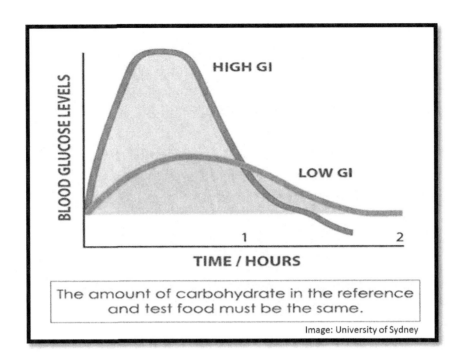

5. **ISO Avail Carb**: This column shows you the ISO assigned Available Carbs for each food in the group. This is the number used to figure out the ISO Glycemic Load (GL) score for each serving. Keep in mind; this is not the same as Total Carbs.

6. **ISO GL**: This is the ISO Glycemic Load (GL) score for the food based on the GI rank and the number of ISO assigned Available Carbs. We can use this as we figure how much of a food we want to eat. Each unit of GL has the same impact on our blood sugar as one gram of Glucose. We can use the ISO GL scores as our guide as we design our own serving sizes to keep our blood sugar levels steady. This way we have our own GL score before we even eat a food.

Glycemic Load Scores:

Low GL = 1-10
Medium GL = 11-19
High GL = 20+

Now when we figure any Glycemic Load (GL) Score, we only count the Available Carbs. That's because these are the Carbs that are available for digestion. This is different than Total Carbs, because Total Carbs include carbs that we cannot even digest. This makes GL far more accurate to manage our blood sugar, as we spoke of earlier.

In the following diagram, you can see that the Glycemic Index (GI) is just as important as the number of Available Carbs in a serving. These two factors come together as they create the Glycemic Load (GL).

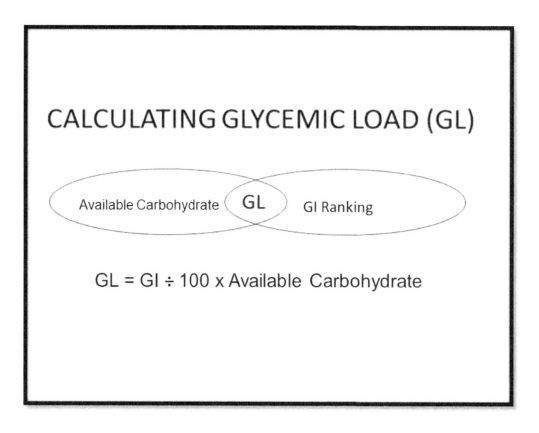

- **Third three columns** come alive with your personal choices. This is your space to experiment until you are satisfied with your result. You may like to use a pencil or add a sticky note for yourself. This way you can try on different serving sizes until you reach your desired Low Glycemic Load Score.

    7. **Your ServSize Oz. /g**.: Enter the amount of the specific food you plan to eat. You may use Metric or Customary US measures as you create a record of your desired serving size.

8. **Your Avail. Carb**: Determine the Avail Carb for your chosen serving size. This is the Total g Carbs in your serving size minus the Fiber g.
   In this column, enter the Available Carbs of the serving size for the food you have selected.

   In other words, the number of Avail Carbs you will have depends on your serving size of that food. Referring to the ISO Avail Carb and ISO GL columns can be quite useful here.

   For example, in the Bakery Products category, you will notice that most Bakery Products have ISO 30g Avail Carb. Based on those ISO 30g Avail Carb, all of the Bakery Products also have a high ISO Glycemic Load, as you see. However, if you went with 15g or 10g Avail Carb instead of the ISO 30g of Avail Carb, you easily arrive at a low GL for most Bakery Products.

   When you decide the number of Available Carbs for your serving size, enter it in the "Your Avail Carbs" column, right after Your Serving Size for that food.

9. **Your GL**: Using the GI information in column 4, and the Your Avail Carb g amount you entered in column 7, calculate Your GL (Glycemic Load). Enter the information in column 8, Your GL. There are several ways to calculate Your GL (Glycemic Load):

   [This might seem repetitive to some of you, but I am including several options to figure Glycemic Load. One person may understand it one way while another person understands it in another way. The important thing is to be sure that everyone who wants to can understand and use this powerful tool.]

   Whichever method you prefer, you will always get the same Glycemic Load (GL) score. A GL score of 10 or less is an ideal low GL score. A low GL score keeps blood sugar within a healthy range.

   GL = GI ÷ 100 x Your Available Carb grams

   We talked earlier about using 5th grade arithmetic. Now, the great thing about this is that it involves the commutative property for multiplication and division.

Commutative is like when you commute to your job; you go from one place to another but you stay the same. In arithmetic, you can move the numbers from one place to another, and the answer comes out the same. How great is that?

I love to be able to tell you that when you have the number of available carbs and the GI ranking, the GL score falls right into your hands. And that is true! It's like a way to "grade" the suitability of your servings.

Here are ways to figure the GL:

GL = GI X Available Carb grams ÷ 100.
GL = Available Carb grams X GI ÷ 100
GL = Carb grams ÷ 100 X GI

On the other hand, maybe it works better for you if you look at it like this:

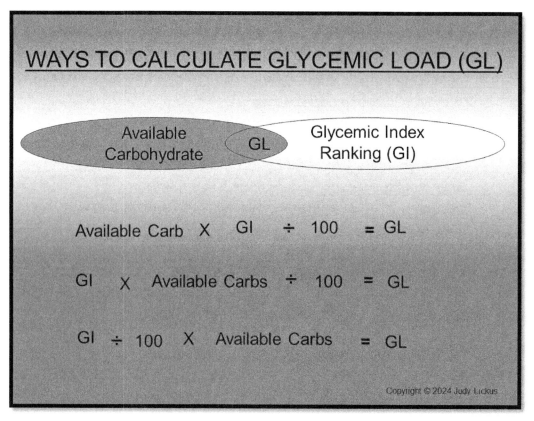

Now, let's do one together, shall we? So for your first food, let's say you have a GI of 50. When you figure GL, you can begin by dividing the GI by

100. And 50 divided by 100 is .5. Next, multiply .5 times the number of Available Carbs you have to get your GL.

So, the GL calculation of a food with a GI of 50 and 20 g of Available Carbs might look like this:

.5 x 20 = 10. 10 or less is a Low Glycemic Load Score.

As you progress through your favorite foods in the Smart Chart Tables™, you will develop a system. Perhaps if you attend the GI first, things may go quicker.

Or, maybe taking 10% of the total after you multiply the GI by the number of Available Carbs is the method that works best for you.

No matter which of the ways you feel most comfortable with, you will arrive at the same answer.

CONGRATULATIONS

Hooray! You did it! You have successfully calculated your first Low GL Score! How wonderful it is that you have a Low GL Score for this serving! ♥

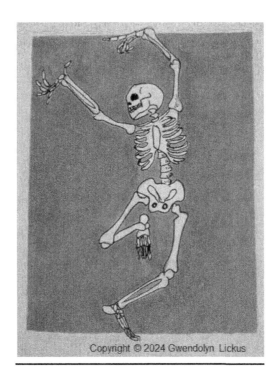

Time for a little "Happy Dance." Now that you have identified your first desirable low GL score, you know the quantity of that food to put on your plate to keep a Low Glycemic Load!

Once you have it, you can use it to figure any food. Nothing or no one can take it away from you.

As you continue to research your favorite foods, you will get better at it, and the work will go much faster. Soon you may find you are able to "do it in your head."

Writing your scores down in the book lets you keep track of what you have learned. No more hunting down loose scraps of paper! You can always check your own personal record. This record will help as you design your own recipes, plan your meals, and maintain your own effective Low Glycemic Load (GL) lifestyle.

As you get going, you may find that the data in the ISO columns can help you figure your way to a low GL even more quickly. Remember, when a 30g carb serving has a GL of 20, cutting the serving size in half gives you a GL of 10. See how that shortcut works? You ARE on the right track. Keep up the good work!

I hope this work pays off for you. You deserve to live the wondrous life that is your natural birthright. Even if this work helps only a few people to better health free from a life of disease and complications, it is worth it to me. I hope it is worth it to you. Out of all the books out there, thank you for reading this one.

Next, the Smart Chart Tables™ begin. I hope they are as helpful as you can expect. Following the Smart Chart Tables™, you will find a few pages for you to keep track of your Troubleshooting and any Meal Prep Notes you may like to keep handy.

BAKERY PRODUCTS ISO 30g AVAIL CARB

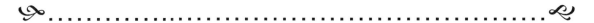

Pub Ref #	ISO Assigned Category	Food & Food Details	GI	ISO Avail Carb	ISO GL	Your Serv Size	Your Avail Carb	Your GL
A1	Bakery	Angel food cake (Loblaw's, Toronto, Canada)	67	30	20			
G/USDA/JL	Bakery	1/12 Angel food cake from recipe in *Are You Sweet Enough Already?*	40	6*	2			
H/USDA	Bakery	Apple muffin, made with rolled oats and without sugar	48	30	14			
H/USDA	Bakery	Apple muffin, made with rolled oats and sugar	44	30	13			
H/USDA	Bakery	Banana cake, made with sugar	47	30	14			
H/USDA	Bakery	Banana cake, made without sugar	55	30	17			
A4/C3	Bakery	Chocolate Cake made from packet mix with chocolate frosting (Betty Crocker General Mills Inc. Minneapolis USA)	38	30	11			
USDA/JL	Bakery	1/12 Recipe Gingerbread Baby-Cakes	55	16*	9			

GLYCEMIC LOAD CARB COUNTER

Pub Ref #	ISO Assigned Category	Food & Food Details	GI	ISO Avail Carb	ISO GL	Your Serv Size	Your Avail Carb	Your GL
		recipe in *Are You Sweet Enough Already?*						
C31b	Bakery	Gingerbread cake, mean of 3 studies, France 2019*	89±8	30	27			
C46	Bakery	Muffin made with oat flour Singapore 2015*	54±5	30	16			
C47	Bakery	Muffin made with barley flour Singapore 2015*	55±5	30	17			
C48	Bakery	Muffin made with corn flour Singapore 2015*	74±5	30	22			
C49	Bakery	Muffin made with wheat flour Singapore 2015*	74±8	30	22			
C50	Bakery	Muffin made with rice flour Singapore 2015*	79±6	30	24			
H/USDA	Bakery	Muffin, 1/12 Chocolate Black Bean Cake, flourless (Recipe in *Are You Sweet Enough Already?)*	40	19*	8			
C54	Bakery	Pancakes, millet (100% foxtail millet flour) China 2016*	76±11	30	23			
C55	Bakery	Pancakes, prepared from	80±4	30	24			

GLYCEMIC LOAD CARB COUNTER

Pub Ref #	ISO Assigned Category	Food & Food Details	GI	ISO Avail Carb	ISO GL	Your Serv Size	Your Avail Carb	Your GL
		wheat flour China 2005						
C68	Bakery	Pizza base, baked in oven at 220°C for 9 min (Boboli, Orograin Bakeries Manufacturing Inc, PA, USA) USA 2015*	52±4	30	16			
H/USDA	Bakery	Sponge cake	46	30	12			
C19	Bakery	Vanilla cake made from packet mix with vanilla frosting (Betty Crocker® USA)	42±4	30	13			
H/USDA/C	Bakery	Waffles, Aunt Jemima®	76	30	23			

BEVERAGES ISO 25g AVAIL CARB

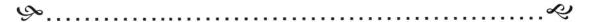

Pub Ref#	ISO Category	Food & Food Details	GI	ISO Avail Carb	ISO GL	Your Serv Size	Your Avail Carb	Your GL
G/USDA	Beverage	Almond Milk, unsweetened, 8 oz./240 mL	0	1*	0			
H	Beverage Fruit Juice	Apple juice, unsweetened	41	20*	8			
A389/USDA	Beverage Fruit Juice	Apple juice, unsweetened (USA)	40	20*	8			
C1184b	Beverage Fruit Juice	Apple juice, mean of five foods (Aus, Ital.)	46	20*	9			
C72	Beverage	*Beer (4.5% alcohol by volume) (Nikolai Lager, Sinebrychoff Ltd, Finland) Finland 2012*	119 ±10	10*	12			
C73	Beverage	*Beer (4.4% alcohol by volume), Pilsner Urquell® (Plzeňský Prazdroj, A.S., Czech Republic)11 Czech Republic 2016*	89±2	10*	9			
C74	Beverage	*Beer, non-alcoholic (0.0% alcohol by volume) (Nikolai Lager, Sinebrychoff Ltd, Finland) Finland 2012*	80±6	10*	8			
C1235	Beverage	*Breast milk, human, unpasteurized Australia 2011* (tested on adults)	38±7	10*	4			

GLYCEMIC LOAD CARB COUNTER

Pub Ref#	ISO Category	Food & Food Details	GI	ISO Avail Carb	ISO GL	Your Serv Size	Your Avail Carb	Your GL
C1190	Beverage Vegetable Juice	Carrot juice, freshly made, Australia	43±3	10*	4			
A21	Beverage	Coca Cola®	63	25	16			
USDA	Beverage	Coconut Milk, unsweetened, 1/3 cup, 2.67 oz./80 mL	40	2*	1			
G	Beverage	Coffee or tea, black, unsweetened	0	0*	0			
A402/C1192	Beverage Fruit Juice	Cranberry juice cocktail (Ocean Spray Inc., USA)	68±3	20*	14			
C1193b	Beverage Fruit Juice	Cranberry juice, mean of three studies (Aus, UK, USA)	59	20*	9			
H	Beverage	Fanta®	68	25	17			
B49	Beverage	Fruit punch (USA)	67	25	17			
H	Beverage	Gatorade®, orange flavor	89	25	22			
C1194	Beverage Fruit Juic	Grape juice, 100%, Daily C (Weichuan Shanghai, China) China 2019*	63±5	20*	13			
B51	Beverage	Mars Active® Energy Drink flavored milk (M&M/Mars USA)	46	25	12			
A416	Beverage Fruit Juice	Orange juice, reconstituted from frozen concentrate (USA)	57	20*	11			
H	Beverage Fruit Juice	Orange juice, unsweetened	50	20*	10			
C1198b	Beverage Fruit Juice	Orange juice, mean of three foods	48	20*	10			
C1199	Beverage Fruit	POM Pomegranate	53±3	20*	11			

GLYCEMIC LOAD CARB COUNTER

Pub Ref#	ISO Category	Food & Food Details	GI	ISO Avail Carb	ISO GL	Your Serv Size	Your Avail Carb	Your GL
	Juice	juice, (POM Wonderful, LLC, USA) 2009*						
G/USDA	Beverage	Seltzer water, baking extract flavored, stevia sweetened	0	0*	0			
B58/C119	Beverage	Smoothie banana & strawberry V8 Splash® (Campbell's Soup Co Camden USA)	44	25	11			
A25/C122	Beverage	Smoothie, raspberry (Con Agra Inc. Omaha USA)	33	25	8			
C135	Beverage	Sport beverage based on whey protein powder with carbohydrate (CHO:PRO=4:1), orange flavor (Endurox R4, Pacific Health Laboratories, Parsippany, NJ, USA) USA 2017*	67±6	25	17			
C1202	Beverage	*Tomato juice, canned, no sugar added (Australia)	38±4	10*	4			
B69/C94	Beverage	V8 Splash® tropical blend fruit drink(Campbell's Soup Company USA)	47	25	9			
B71	Beverage	V8® 100% vegetable juice (Campbell's Soup Company USA)	43	20*	9			
USDA/G	Beverage	Water; plain, tap, bottled,	0	0*	0			

GLYCEMIC LOAD CARB COUNTER

Pub Ref#	ISO Category	Food & Food Details	GI	ISO Avail Carb	ISO GL	Your Serv Size	Your Avail Carb	Your GL
		carbonated, unsweetened						

GLYCEMIC LOAD CARB COUNTER

BREAD & RICE CAKES ISO 15g AVAIL CARB

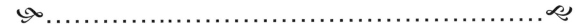

Pub Ref #	ISO Category	Food & Food Details	GI	ISO 15 g Avail Carb	ISO GL	Your Serv Size	Your Avail Carb	Your GL
A143	Bread	100% Whole Grain™ (Natural Ovens USA)	51	15	8			
H	Bread	50% cracked wheat kernel	58	15	9			
C875	Bread	9 Grain cracker Australia 2013*	68±5	15	10			
B101	Bread	Bagel white (USA)	69	15	10			
H	Bread	Bagel, white, frozen	72	15	11			
H	Bread	Baguette, white, plain	93	15	14			
C736	Bread	Biscuit, wholegrain USA 2018*	54±5	15	8			
C737	Bread	Biscuits, wholegrain, filled with peanut butter USA 2018*	44±3	15	7			
H	Bread	Coarse barley bread, 80% kernels	34	15	5			
C328	Bread	Corn tortilla, made from white corn, gluten-free, Mission® Foods, Australia 2010*	52±4	15	8			
A121/C145	Bread	English Muffin™ bread (Natural Ovens USA)	77	15	12			

41

GLYCEMIC LOAD CARB COUNTER

Pub Ref #	ISO Category	Food & Food Details	GI	ISO 15 g Avail Carb	ISO GL	Your Serv Size	Your Avail Carb	Your GL
C158b	Bread	Fruit bread, mean of 12 foods	57	15	9			
C163b	Bread	Gluten-free breads, mean of five foods	59	15	9			
H	Bread	Hamburger bun	61	15	9			
A71/C155	Bread	Happiness™ (cinnamon raisin pecan bread) (Natural Ovens Manitowoc USA)	63	15	9			
A123/C172	Bread	Healthy Choice™ Hearty 100% Whole Grain (Con Agra Inc. USA)	62	15	9			
A122/C171	Bread	Healthy Choice™ Hearty 7 Grain (Con Agra Inc. USA)	55	15	8			
A126/C192	Bread	Hunger Filler™ whole grain bread (Natural Ovens USA)	59	15	9			
H/USDA	Bread	Kaiser roll	73	15	11			
C198	Bread	Lower Carb 5 Seeds Bread, Helga's™ (Quality Bakers, Sydney, Australia) Australia 2018*	53±5	15	8			

GLYCEMIC LOAD CARB COUNTER

Pub Ref #	ISO Category	Food & Food Details	GI	ISO 15 g Avail Carb	ISO GL	Your Serv Size	Your Avail Carb	Your GL
C196b	Bread	Mixed grain or seed bread, mean of 27 foods	56	15	8			
C200b	Bread	Mixed grain or seed wheat bread, lower carbohydrate mean of four foods	45	15	7			
C330	Bread	Mixed Grain wraps, Helga's (Quality Bakers Australia Pty Ltd,) Australia 2015*	55±6	15	8			
A72	Bread	Muesli bread made from packet mix in bread making machine (Con Agra Inc. USA)	54	15	8			
A131/C193	Bread	Nutty Natural™ whole grain bread (Natural Ovens USA)	59	15	9			
C206b	Bread	Oatmeal batch breads, mean of six foods	65	15	10			
H/USDA	Bread	Pita bread, white	68	15	10			
C329	Bread	Protein Wraps (Herman Brot Pty Ltd.) Australia 2019*	27±3	15	4			

GLYCEMIC LOAD CARB COUNTER

Pub Ref #	ISO Category	Food & Food Details	GI	ISO 15 g Avail Carb	ISO GL	Your Serv Size	Your Avail Carb	Your GL
C882	Rice Cake	Puffed Rice Cake, caramel flavored, USA	82±10	15	12			
H/USDA	Bread	Pumpernickel	56	15	8			
C216	Bread	Pumpernickel Rye bread (Van der Meulen BV.) Netherlands 2015*	49±4	15	7			
C224b	Bread	Rye breads, mean of 13 foods	60	15	9			
C207	Bread	Soft pretzel, soy USA 2011*	39±6	15	6			
C208	Bread	Soft pretzel, wheat USA 2011*	66±4	15	10			
C227	Bread	Sourdough bread (50% wholemeal wheat, 50% white wheat, sourdough starter (70% wet weight), 80 min rising time, 60 min proving time, 200°C baking temperature, 60 min baking time13 New Zealand 2010*	82±13	15	12			

Pub Ref #	ISO Category	Food & Food Details	GI	ISO 15 g Avail Carb	ISO GL	Your Serv Size	Your Avail Carb	Your GL
C228	Bread	Sourdough bread + oats (50% wholemeal wheat, 50% white wheat, 10% rolled oats; sourdough starter (70% wet weight), 80 min rising time, 60 min proving time, 200°C baking temperature, 60 min baking time13 New Zealand 2010*	71±10	15	11			
C220	Bread	Sourdough bread, made with rye flour, wholemeal rye flour, spelt flour and intact barley kernels and white bean kernels Sweden 2020*	67±5	15	10			
C221	Bread	Sourdough bread, made with rye flour, wholemeal rye flour, spelt flour with intact barley kernels and mung bean kernels Sweden 2020*	65±4	15	10			

GLYCEMIC LOAD CARB COUNTER

Pub Ref #	ISO Category	Food & Food Details	GI	ISO 15 g Avail Carb	ISO GL	Your Serv Size	Your Avail Carb	Your GL
C229b	Bread	Sourdough wheat breads, mean of five foods	70	15	11			
A137/C	Bread	Soy & Linseed bread (made from packet mix cooked in bread maker) (Con Agra Inc. USA)	50	15	8			
C223b		Spelt bread, mean of four foods	61	15	9			
A138/C194	Bread	Stay Trim™ whole grain bread (Natural Ovens USA)	70	15	11			
C236/Pkg.	Bread	White bread (Giant Eagle King Size Enriched bread, Pittsburgh, PA, USA) USA 2011*	60±6	15	9			
C237/Pkg.	Bread	White bread (Pepperidge Farm Original White Bread, USA) USA 2016*	62±2	15	9			
C268b	Bread	White wheat flour bread, mean of 35 foods	73	15	11			

GLYCEMIC LOAD CARB COUNTER

Pub Ref #	ISO Category	Food & Food Details	GI	ISO 15 g Avail Carb	ISO GL	Your Serv Size	Your Avail Carb	Your GL
B177	Bread	White wheat flour bread, white flour (Pepperidge Farm Norwalk CT USA)	71	15	11			
H/USDA	Bread	White wheat flour bread, average	75	15	11			
A101	Bread	White-wheat-flour bread (USA)	70	15	11			
C332	Bread	Whole Grain Tortilla, Old El Paso™ (General Mills) Australia 2015*	50±5	15	8			
H/USDA	Bread	Whole wheat, average	71	15	12			
A116/USDA	Bread	Whole-meal (whole-wheat) wheat-flour bread Whole-meal flour (USA)	73	15	11			
C333	Bread	Wholemeal and white flour wrap with chia seeds, Mission™ brand (Gruma Oceania Pty Ltd.) Australia* 2015*	50±6	15	8			

GLYCEMIC LOAD CARB COUNTER

Pub Ref #	ISO Category	Food & Food Details	GI	ISO 15 g Avail Carb	ISO GL	Your Serv Size	Your Avail Carb	Your GL
C334	Bread	Wholemeal and white flour wrap with red quinoa, Mission™ brand (Gruma Oceania Pty Ltd.) Australia 2015*	59±5	15	9			
C322b	Bread	Wholemeal wheat flour bread, mean of eight foods	75	15	12			
A103/Pkg	Bread	Wonder, enriched white bread (Interstate Brands Companies, Kansas City, MO, USA) Mean of 3 studies	73	15	11			
B197/Pkg	Bread	Wonder® bread, average	73	15	11			
B196	Bread	Wonder™ enriched white bread	72	15	11			

GLYCEMIC LOAD CARB COUNTER

BREAKFAST CEREALS & COOKIES ISO 20g AVAIL CARB

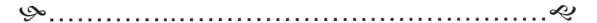

Pub Ref #	ISO Category	Food & Food Details	GI	ISO 20 g Avail Carb	ISO GL	Your Serv Size	Your Avail Carb	Your GL
A151	Breakfast Cereal	All-Bran® (high-fiber, extruded wheat-bran cereal) (Kellogg's, Battle Creek, MI, USA)	38	20	8			
B299	Breakfast Cereal	All-Bran®, average	55	20	11			
C736	Cookie	Biscuit, wholegrain USA 2018*	54±5	20	11			
C737	Cookie	Biscuits, wholegrain, filled with peanut butter USA 2018*	44±3	20	9			
C361b	Breakfast Cereal	Bran flakes, mean of three foods	63	20	13			
C521b	Breakfast Cereal	Breakfast cereal bars, mean of 16 foods	56	20	11			
A168	Breakfast Cereal	Cornflakes (Kellogg's, USA)	92	20	19			
C374b	Breakfast Cereal	Cornflakes, mean of 10 foods	80	20	16			
H	Breakfast Cereal	Cornflakes®, average	81	20	16			
C388b	Breakfast Cereal	Granola, mean of 11 foods	53	20	11			
C381	Breakfast Cereal	Granola, whole-grain oat protein USA 2018*	51±4	20	10			

GLYCEMIC LOAD CARB COUNTER

Pub Ref #	ISO Category	Food & Food Details	GI	ISO 20 g Avail Carb	ISO GL	Your Serv Size	Your Avail Carb	Your GL
A182/B339/C483	Breakfast Cereal	Grapenuts™ (Kraft Foods Inc., Port Chester, NY, USA)	75	20	15			
B346	Breakfast Cereal	Hot cereal apple & cinnamon (Con Agra Inc., USA)	37	20	7			
B347	Breakfast Cereal	Hot cereal unflavored (Con Agra Inc., USA)	25	20	5			
A189	Breakfast Cereal	Hot cereal, apple and cinnamon (Con Agra Inc., USA)	37	20	7			
A190	Breakfast Cereal	Hot cereal, unflavored (Con Agra Inc., USA)	25	20	5			
B350	Breakfast Cereal	Kashi Seven Whole Grain Puffs®	65	20	13			
C422b	Breakfast Cereal	Muesli, mean of 30 foods	55	20	11			
C429b	Breakfast Cereal	Oats, Instant oat porridge, mean of four foods	82	20	16			
H	Breakfast Cereal	Oats, instant, average, one packet (41g)	79	20	16			
H/USDA/C	Breakfast Cereal	Oats, Oatmeal average	55	20	11			
C427b	Breakfast Cereals	Oats, Porridge made from rolled oats, mean of eight foods	58	20	12			
C442b	Breakfast Cereal	Oats, Porridge made from	52	20	10			

GLYCEMIC LOAD CARB COUNTER

Pub Ref #	ISO Category	Food & Food Details	GI	ISO 20 g Avail Carb	ISO GL	Your Serv Size	Your Avail Carb	Your GL
		steel-cut oats, mean of 5 foods						
B390/C	Breakfast Cereal	Oats, Porridge make from steel cut oats boiled in water	52	20	10			
C422	Breakfast Cereal	Oats, Whole-grain oat muesli USA 2018*	55±4	20	11			
A220/B414/C500	Breakfast Cereal	Raisin Bran ™ (Kellogg's, USA)	61	20	12			
A228/B423/C448	Breakfast Cereal	Special K™ (Kellogg's, USA)	69	20	14			
C505	Breakfast Cereal	Whole-grain protein cereal USA 2018*	49±3	20	10			

CEREAL GRAINS ISO 45g AVAIL CARB

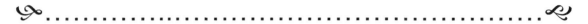

Pub Ref #	ISO Category	Food & Food Details	GI	ISO 45 g Avail Carb	ISO GL	Your Serv Size	Your Avail Carb	Your GL
C546	Cereal Grain	Barley, AC Parkhill cultivar (two-rowed, hulled, normal barley; high amylose, low ß-glucan) white pearled (all of the bran and most of the germ and crease removed), boiled for 30 min Canada 2012*	41±5	45	18			
C547b	Cereal Grain	Barley, mean of 20 foods	30	45	14			
H	Cereal Grain	Barley, pearled, average	25	45	11			
C553b	Cereal Grain	Barley, Porridge made from barley, mean of four studies	44	45	20			
C543	Cereal Grain	Barley, pot, boiled (Goudas Food Products, Canada) Canada 2001	35±4	45	16			
H	Cereal Grain	Bulgur, average, cooked	47	45	21			
G/USDA	Grain/ Alternative	Flour, Almond flour, 2 Tbsp./15 g	0	1*	0			
G/USDA	Grain/ Alternative	Flour, Chickpea	10	5*	1			

GLYCEMIC LOAD CARB COUNTER

Pub Ref #	ISO Category	Food & Food Details	GI	ISO 45 g Avail Carb	ISO GL	Your Serv Size	Your Avail Carb	Your GL
		flour, 2 Tbsp./15 g						
B1171/USDA	Grain/ Alternative	Flour, Coconut flour, 2 Tbsp./15 g.	42	4*	2			
USDA	Cereal Grain	Flour, Unbleached Wheat, 2 Tbsp./15g	42±2	23*	10			
C705	Cereal Grain	Flour, Whole wheat powder China 2005	42±2	45	19			
C616b	Cereal Grain	Jasmine rice, white, mean of 18 studies	89	45	40			
C555	Cereal Grain	Polenta, Cornmeal porridge China 2005	68±3	45	31			
H	Cereal Grain	Quinoa	53	45	24			
C571b	Cereal Grain	Quinoa, mean of four foods	53	45	24			
C634b	Cereal Grain	Rice long grain, mean of six foods	62	45	28			
C583b	Cereal Grain	Rice, Basmati rice, white, mean of 10 studies	60	45	27			
C591b	Cereal Grain	Rice, Basmati, quick cooking, mean of four foods	65	45	29			
B535/C626	Cereal Grain	Rice, Brown & Wild Uncle Ben's® Ready Whole Grain Medley™ (pouch) (Effem Foods USA)	45	45	20			
B534/625	Cereal Grain	Rice, Brown Rice Uncle Ben's® Ready Whole Grain (pouch)	48	45	22			

GLYCEMIC LOAD CARB COUNTER

Pub Ref #	ISO Category	Food & Food Details	GI	ISO 45 g Avail Carb	ISO GL	Your Serv Size	Your Avail Carb	Your GL
		(Effem Foods USA)						
A298	Cereal Grain	Rice, Brown, steamed (USA)	50	45	23			
B536/C627	Cereal Grain	Rice, Chicken Flavored Brown Rice Uncle Ben's® Ready Whole Grain (pouch) (Effem Foods USA)	46	45	21			
B603	Cereal Grain	Rice, Converted, white boiled 20-30 min Uncle Ben's® (Masterfoods USA)	38	45	17			
A300	Cereal Grain	Rice, Converted, white, boiled 20-30 min (Uncle Ben's®; Masterfoods USA, Vernon, CA)	38	45	17			
A300	Cereal Grain	Rice, Converted, white, long grain, boiled 20-30 min (Uncle Ben's®; Masterfoods USA)	50	45	23			
C598b	Cereal Grain	Rice, Doongara rice, mean of seven studies	54	45	24			
C647b	Cereal Grain	Rice, Instant white rice, mean of 12 foods	60	45	27			

GLYCEMIC LOAD CARB COUNTER

Pub Ref #	ISO Category	Food & Food Details	GI	ISO 45 g Avail Carb	ISO GL	Your Serv Size	Your Avail Carb	Your GL
C628b	Cereal Grain	Rice, Instant, brown, mean of four foods	50	45	23			
C613	Cereal Grain	Rice, Jasmine rice, Jazzmen, cooked in rice cooker (Jazzmen Rice, Inc., USA) 11 USA 2014*	106±13	45	48			
B540/C644	Cereal Grain	Rice, Long Grain and Wild Uncle Ben's® Ready Rice (pouch) (Effem Foods USA)	49	45	22			
B542/C645	Cereal Grain	Rice, Original Long Grain Uncle Ben's® Ready Rice (pouch) (Effem Foods USA)	48	45	22			
A300	Cereal Grain	Rice, Parboiled (USA)	72	45	32			
C700b	Cereal Grain	Rice, Parboiled rice, mean of 10 studies	64	45	29			
B544/C679	Cereal Grain	Rice, Roasted Chicken Flavored Uncle Ben's® Ready (pouch) (Effem Foods USA)	51	45	23			
B545/C680	Cereal Grain	Rice, Santa Fe Uncle Ben's® Ready Whole Grain Medley™ (pouch) (Effem Foods USA)	48	45	22			

GLYCEMIC LOAD CARB COUNTER

Pub Ref #	ISO Category	Food & Food Details	GI	ISO 45 g Avail Carb	ISO GL	Your Serv Size	Your Avail Carb	Your GL
B546/C681	Cereal Grain	Rice, Spanish Style Uncle Ben's® Ready Rice (pouch) (Effem Foods USA)	51	45	23			
B547/C687	Cereal Grain	Rice, Vegetable Harvest Uncle Ben's® Ready Whole Grain Medley™ (pouch) (Effem Foods USA)	48	45	22			
H	Cereal Grain	Rice, White rice, boiled, type non-specified	72	45	32			
C591b	Cereal Grain	Rice, white, quick cooking Basmati, mean of 4 foods	65	45	29			
B504	Cereal Grain	Sweet corn	60	45	27			
A265	Cereal Grain	Sweet corn (USA)	60	45	27			
H	Cereal Grain	Sweet corn on the cob	48	45	22			
B1619	Cereal Grain	Sweet corn, boiled	60	45	27			
A597	Cereal Grain	Sweet corn, whole-kernel, diet pack, Featherweight, canned, drained, heated, USA	46	45	21			

GLYCEMIC LOAD CARB COUNTER

DAIRY & ALTERNATIVES ISO 20g AVAIL CARB

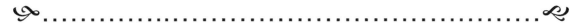

Pub Ref #	ISO Category	Food & Food Details	GI	ISO Avail Carb	ISO GL	Your Serv Size	Your Avail Carb	Your GL
G/USDA	Dairy Alternative	Almond Milk, unsweetened, 8 oz./240 mL	0	1*	0			
C1235*	Dairy, Infant foods	Breast milk, human, unpasteurized Australia 2011* (tested on adults)	38±7	10*	4*			
USDA	Dairy Alternative	Coconut Milk, unsweetened, 1/3 cup, 2.67 oz./80 mL	40	2*	1			
C922	Dairy	Ice cream, low-fat, Dutch Chocolate flavor (ProYo, USA) USA 2017*	34±6	20	7			
C923	Dairy	Ice cream, low-fat, Mint Chip flavor (ProYo, USA) USA 2017*	34±6	20	7			
C924	Dairy	Ice cream, low-fat, Mocha flavor (ProYo, USA) USA 2017*	37±5	20	7			
C925	Dairy	Ice cream, low-fat, Vanilla Bean flavor (ProYo, USA) USA 2017*	39±5	20	8			
H	Dairy	Ice cream, premium (Sara Lee®)	38	20	8			
H	Dairy	Ice cream, regular, average	62	20	12			
C925b	Dairy	Ice-cream, reduced- or	36	20	7			

Pub Ref #	ISO Category	Food & Food Details	GI	ISO Avail Carb	ISO GL	Your Serv Size	Your Avail Carb	Your GL
		low-fat, mean of 17 foods						
C934	Dairy	Kefir, low-fat strawberry (Lifeway Foods, Chicago, USA) USA 2012*	60±10	20	12			
C933	Dairy	Kefir, low-fat, plain (Lifeway Foods, Chicago, USA) USA 2012*	36±9	20	7			
C935	Dairy	Kefir, orange flavor (Lifeway Foods, Chicago, USA) USA 2012*	48±10	20	10			
C939b	Dairy	Milk, full-fat, mean of 3 foods	37	10*	4			
C954b	Dairy	Milk, reduced- or low-fat, flavored, mean of 7 foods	29	20	6			
C947b	Dairy	Milk, Reduced-fat or low-fat milk, mean of 6 foods	27	10*	3			
B816	Dairy	Milk, skim (USA)	32	10*	3			
H	Dairy	Milk, skim, average	31	10*	3			
C964b	Dairy	Mousse, reduced-fat, commercially prepared mix prepared with water, mean of 9 foods	38	20	8			
C967b	Dairy	Pudding, Flavored milk pudding, made with whole milk, mean of 3 foods	46	20	9			

GLYCEMIC LOAD CARB COUNTER

Pub Ref #	ISO Category	Food & Food Details	GI	ISO Avail Carb	ISO GL	Your Serv Size	Your Avail Carb	Your GL
C1068b	Dairy	Soy milk full-fat, mean of 5 foods	37	20	7			
C1072b	Dairy	Soy milk reduced-fat, mean of 4 foods	31	20	6			
A387	Dairy	Tofu-based frozen dessert, chocolate with high fructose (24%) corn syrup (USA)	115	20	23			
C1002b	Dairy	Yoghurt, different flavors, mean of 25 foods	35	20	7			
C1030b	Dairy	Yoghurt, Low fat yoghurts different flavors, mean of 25 foods	32	20	6			
C1027	Dairy	Yoghurt, Low-fat, sugar sweetened, Passionfruit flavor, Vaalia (Pauls Ltd) Australia	32±3	20	6			
C1046	Dairy	Yoghurt, No Added Sugar Natural yoghurt (Tamar Valley Dairy, Australia) Australia 2010*	17±2	10*	2			
C1029	Dairy	Yoghurt, No Added Sugar Passionfruit, Tamar Valley (Aldi, Australia) 2010*	21±2	20	4			
C1045b	Dairy	Yoghurt, Non-fat yoghurts, mean of 7 foods	26	20	5			

GLYCEMIC LOAD CARB COUNTER

Pub Ref #	ISO Category	Food & Food Details	GI	ISO Avail Carb	ISO GL	Your Serv Size	Your Avail Carb	Your GL
C1038b	Dairy	Yoghurt, Reduced-fat Yoghurts different flavors, mean of 9 foods	30	20	6			
C1049b	Dairy	Yoghurts, All Yoghurts, mean of 72 foods	33	20	7			
H	Dairy	Yoghurt, Reduced-fat yogurt with fruit, average	33	20	7			

FRUIT and FRUIT PRODUCTS ISO 15g AVAIL CARB

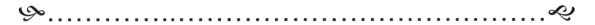

Pub Ref #	ISO Category	Food & Food Details	GI	ISO Carb	ISO GL	Your Serv Size	Your Avail Carb	Your GL
C1184b	Fruit Juice	Apple juice, mean of five foods (Aus, Ital.)	46	20*	9			
H	Fruit Juice	Apple juice, unsweetened	41	20*	8			
A389/USDA	Fruit Juice	Apple juice, unsweetened (USA)	40	20*	8			
A388	Fruit	Apples, raw, NS (USA)	40	15	6			
C1208	Fruit Product	Apricot 100% Fruit Spread, Cottees™ (Cadbury Schweppes, Australia) Australia 2004	50±6	15	8			
C1213	Fruit Product	Apricot jam (Confettura extra albicocche, Bonne Maman, Italy) Italy 2010*	69±6	15	10			
C1213b	Fruit Product	Apricot spread, mean of seven foods 57	57	15	9			
G	Fruit	Avocado	0		0			
C1749b		Banana, Green banana, mean of five foods	39	15	6			
A397k	Fruit	Banana, mean of 10 foods	52±4	15	8			
A397i	Fruit	Banana, overripe, yellow flecked with brown (USA)	48	15	7			
A397f	Fruit	Banana, raw, ripe, all yellow (USA)	51	15	8			
A397h	Fruit	Banana, slightly under-ripe, yellow with	42	15	6			

Pub Ref #	ISO Category	Food & Food Details	GI	ISO Carb	ISO GL	Your Serv Size	Your Avail Carb	Your GL
		green sections (USA)						
G/#	Fruit	Blackberries	0	15	0			
C1215		Blackberry 100% Fruit Spread, Cottees™ brand (Cadbury Schweppes, Australia) Australia 2004	46±5	15	7			
G	Fruit	Blueberries	29	15	4			
C1216	Fruit Product	Blueberry fruit spread, wild blueberry (Rhapsodie de Fruit Wild Blueberry, St. Dalfour, Italy) Italy 2010*	74±5	15	11			
C1217	Fruit Product	Blueberry jam, wild blueberry (Confettura extra mirtilli selvatici, Bonne Maman, Italy) Italy 2010*	63±3	15	9			
G/#	Fruit	Boysenberries	40	15	6			
G/#	Fruit	Cantaloupe	40	15	6			
G/#	Fruit	Cherries, red	40	15	6			
G/#	Fruit	Cranberries	40	15	6			
C1096		Cranberries, sweetened, dried (Ocean Spray, USA) USA 2011*	62±6	15	9			
A402/C1192	Fruit Juice	Cranberry juice cocktail (Ocean Spray Inc., USA)	68±3	20*	14			
C1193b	Fruit Juice	Cranberry juice, mean of three studies (Aus, UK, USA)	59	20*	9			
H	Fruit	Dates	42	15	6			

GLYCEMIC LOAD CARB COUNTER

Pub Ref #	ISO Category	Food & Food Details	GI	ISO Carb	ISO GL	Your Serv Size	Your Avail Carb	Your GL
C1128b	Fruit	Dates, dried, mean of 19 foods	54	15	8			
C1109b	Fruit	Dates, mean of 11 foods	52	15	8			
C1128b	Fruit	Dates, mean of 19 foods	54	15	8			
C3017	Fruit	Dragon fruit/Pitahaya (Hylocereus spp.), pulp, raw, frozen, thawed Costa Rica 2012*	48±11	15	7			
G/#	Fruit	Figs	40	15	6			
C1129	Fruit	Figs, dried, no added, sugar, organic, Turkish (Woolworths Macro brand, Australia) Turkey 2018*	54±6	15	8			
C1129	Fruit	Figs, dried, no added, sugar, organic, Turkish (Woolworths Macro brand, Australia) Turkey 2018*	54±6	15	8			
C1194	Fruit Juice	Grape juice, 100%, Daily C (Weichuan Shanghai, China) China 2019*	63±5	20*	13			
H	Fruit	Grapefruit	25	15	4			
H	Fruit	Grapes, Black	59	15	9			
G/#	Fruit	Guava	40	15	6			
C1131	Fruit	Guava, raw, cut into bite size pieces Singapore 2017*	29±4	15	4			
C1132	Fruit	Guava, raw, puree Singapore 2017*	47±4	15	7			
G/#	Fruit	Honeydew	40	15	6			

GLYCEMIC LOAD CARB COUNTER

Pub Ref #	ISO Category	Food & Food Details	GI	ISO Carb	ISO GL	Your Serv Size	Your Avail Carb	Your GL
C1095		Jackfruit, Green Jackfruit, prepared as a porridge with water India 2016*	65±5	15	10			
G/#	Fruit	Kiwi	40	15	6			
G/#	Fruit	Lychee	40	15	6			
C1138		Lychee, fresh Australia 2009*	57±3	15	9			
G/#	Fruit	Mandarin	40	15	6			
G/#	Fruit	Mango	40	15	6			
C1142	Fruit	Mango, raw (Chin-Hwang Mango) Taiwan 2010*	48±0.3	15	7			
G/#	Fruit	Mulberries	40	15	6			
C1222	Fruit Product	Orange fruit spread, with thick cut orange (Rhapsodie de Fruit Orange Spread, Thick Cut St Dalfour, Italy) Italy 2010*	68±6	15	10			
C1223	Fruit Product	Orange jam, organic bitter orange, with apple juice (Fiordifrutta arance amare, Rigoni di Asiago, Italy) Italy 2010*	51±8	15	8			
C1198b	Fruit Juice	Orange juice, mean of three foods	48	20*	10			
A416	Fruit Juice	Orange juice, reconstituted from frozen concentrate (USA)	57	20*	11			
H	Fruit Juice	Orange juice, unsweetened	50	20*	10			

GLYCEMIC LOAD CARB COUNTER

Pub Ref #	ISO Category	Food & Food Details	GI	ISO Carb	ISO GL	Your Serv Size	Your Avail Carb	Your GL
C1224	Fruit Product	Orange marmalade, bitter orange (Marmellata arance amare, Bonne Maman, Italy) Italy 2010*	55±6	15	8			
C1227b	Fruit Product	Orange marmalade, mean of six foods	51	15	8			
C1225	Fruit Product	Orange marmalade, orange 100% Pure Fruit spread, no added sugar (Freedom Foods, Australia) Australia 2006	27±3	15	4			
H	Fruit	Orange, raw, average	45	15	7			
A415	Fruit	Oranges, raw (Sunkist, Van Nuys, CA, USA)	48	15	7			
G/#	Fruit	Papaya	40	15	6			
C1153	Fruit	Papaya/paw paw, raw, cut into bite size pieces Singapore 2017*	38±2	15	6			
C1154	Fruit	Papaya/paw paw, raw, puree Singapore 2017*	42±5	15	6			
G/#	Fruit	Passionfruit	40	15	6			
H	Fruit	Peach, average	42	15	6			
H	Fruit	Peach, canned in light syrup	52	15	8			
G	Fruit	Peaches, Delmonte® canned in light syrup (Produced in Canada)	52	15	8			
H	Fruit	Pear	38	15	6			

GLYCEMIC LOAD CARB COUNTER

Pub Ref #	ISO Category	Food & Food Details	GI	ISO Carb	ISO GL	Your Serv Size	Your Avail Carb	Your GL
H	Fruit	Pear, canned in pear juice	44	15	7			
G/#	Fruit	Persimmon	40	15	6			
G/#	Fruit	Pineapple	40	15	6			
G/#	Fruit	Plantain	40	15	6			
G/#	Fruit	Plum	40	15	6			
C1199	Fruit Juice	POM Pomegranate juice (POM Wonderful LLC, USA) USA 2009*	53±3	20*	11			
G/#	Fruit	Pomegranate	40	15	6			
C3021	Fruit	Pomelo, Majia variety (Citrus grandis cv. Majiayou), Fresh (T2D test subjects) China 2013*	72±2	15	11			
C3022	Fruit	Pomelo, Majia variety (Citrus grandis cv. Majiayou), Fresh (Normal test subjects) China 2013*	78±2	15	12			
A433	Fruit	Prunes, pitted (Sunsweet Growers Inc., Yuba City, CA, USA) 2002	29	15	4			
C1169	Fruit	Prunes, pitted, Californian (Sunsweet Growers Inc., Yuba City, USA) USA 2009*	40±6	15	6			
C1799	Fruit	Pumpkin, Butternut pumpkin, boiled Australia 2006	51±6	10*	5*			
H	Fruit	Raisins	64	15	10			
C1173	Fruit	Raisins USA 2009*	61±4	15	10			

Pub Ref #	ISO Category	Food & Food Details	GI	ISO Carb	ISO GL	Your Serv Size	Your Avail Carb	Your GL
C1170	Fruit	Raisins (Sun Maid, USA) USA 2013*	49±4	15	7			
C1173b	Fruit	Raisins, mean of four studies	55	15	8			
G	Fruit	Raspberries	0	15	0			
C1230	Fruit Product	Raspberry 100% Fruit Spread, Cottees™ brand (Cadbury Schweppes, Australia) Australia 2004	46±5	15	7			
C1229	Fruit Product	Raspberry 100% Pure Fruit spread, no added sugar (Freedom Foods, Australia) Australia 2006	26±4	15	4			
G/#	Fruit	Rhubarb	40	15	6			
G/#	Fruit	Rose hips	40	15	6			
G/#	Fruit	Soursop	40	15	6			
G/#	Fruit	Strawberries	40	15	6			
C1232	Fruit Product	Strawberry 100% Pure Fruit spread, no added sugar (Freedom Foods, Australia) Australia 2006	29±4	15	4			
C1231	Fruit Product	Strawberry jam Australia 1998	51±10	15	8			
C1233	Fruit Product	Strawberry 100% Fruit Spread, Cottees™ brand (Cadbury Schweppes, Australia) Australia 2004	46±5	15	7			
C1176	Fruit	Sultanas Canada 2018*	51±4	15	8			
C1544b	Fruit Product	Sweet strawberry fruit	27	15	4			

GLYCEMIC LOAD CARB COUNTER

Pub Ref #	ISO Category	Food & Food Details	GI	ISO Carb	ISO GL	Your Serv Size	Your Avail Carb	Your GL
		leather, Stretch Island, USA, mean of 3 foods						
G/#	Fruit	Tangerine	40	15	6			
G	Fruit	Tomato (Solanum lycopersicum), raw	23	15	3			
B1058	Fruit Juice	Tomato juice, canned	38	10*	4			
C1202	Fruit Juice	Tomato juice, canned, no added sugar (Berri Ltd, Australia)	38±4	10*	4			
H	Fruit	Watermelon	72	15	11			
C1148b	Fruit	Watermelon, mean of 4 foods Malaysia 2017*	50	15	8			

LEGUMES ISO 15g AVAIL CARB

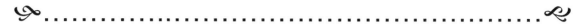

Pub Ref #	ISO Category	Food & Food Details	GI	ISO Avail Carb	ISO GL	Your Serv Size	Your Avail Carb	Your GL
H	Legumes	Beans, baked	40	15	6			
C1283b	Legumes	Beans, Baked Beans, mean of 6 foods	48	15	7			
A571	Legumes	Beans, Black bean (Wil-Pack Foods, San Pedro, CA, USA)	64	15	10			
G	Legumes	Black beans, boiled	31	15	5			
G#	Legumes	Carob bean powder, unsweetened	40	15	6			
G	Legumes	Chickpeas (Cicer arietinum Linn), dried, soaked, boiled 35 min	10	15	2			
G	Legumes	Chickpeas (Garbanzo beans, Bengal gram), canned, drained, Edgell's™ brand	38	15	6			
H	Legumes	Chickpeas, boiled	10	15	2			
G	Legumes	Chickpeas, canned in brine	43	15	6			
C1284	Legumes	Chickpeas, canned, drained (Edgell, Simplot Australia) 2018*	35±3	15	5			

GLYCEMIC LOAD CARB COUNTER

Pub Ref #	ISO Category	Food & Food Details	GI	ISO Avail Carb	ISO GL	Your Serv Size	Your Avail Carb	Your GL
G#	Legumes	Cocoa bean powder, unsweetened	40	15	6			
C1288	Legumes	Hummus (Sabra Classic Hummus; Sabra Dipping Co., S. Chesterfield, VA) USA 2016*	15±3	15	2			
G	Legumes	Kidney beans (Phaseolus vulgaris L.), soaked overnight, boiled, cooled overnight, microwaved	13	15	2			
H	Legumes	Kidney beans, boiled	34	15	5			
G	Legumes	Kidney beans, boiled in salted water	32	15	5			
G	Legumes	Kidney beans, canned (Lancia-Bravo Foods Ltd., Canada)	53	15	8			
C1298b	Legumes	Lentils, washed, brought to boil in water (1:2.5 seed:water ratio) at 500°C (~11 min), once boiling was achieved temperature reduced to 280°C and continued to boil until soft (Saskatchewa	16	15	3			

GLYCEMIC LOAD CARB COUNTER

Pub Ref #	ISO Category	Food & Food Details	GI	ISO Avail Carb	ISO GL	Your Serv Size	Your Avail Carb	Your GL
		n Pulse Growers, Canada) Canada 2017* Mean of 8 foods						
C1298b	Legumes	Lentils, boiled, mean of 8 foods	16	15	2			
H	Legumes	Lentils, cooked	29	15	4			
A462	Legumes	Lentils, type NS Lentils, type NS (USA)	28	15	4			
H	Legumes	Navy beans, average, boiled	39	15	6			
G	Legumes	Pinto beans, boiled in salted water	14	15	2			
G	Legumes	Pinto beans, canned in brine (Lancia-Bravo Foods Ltd., Canada)	45	15	7			
G	Legumes	Pinto beans, dried, boiled	39	15	6			
G	Legumes	Pinto beans, Refried, Casa Fiesta™ brand, heated in microwave for 1.5 min	38	15	6			
G	Legumes	Pinto beans, steamed	33	15	5			
H	Legumes	Soy Beans, boiled	15	15	2			

GLYCEMIC LOAD CARB COUNTER

MEAL REPLACEMENT & WEIGHT MANAGEMENT ISO 20g AVAIL CARB

Pub Ref f#	ISO Category	Food & Food Details	GI	ISO Avail Carb	ISO GL	Your Serv Size	Your Avail Carb	Your GL
B1130	Meal Repl. & Weight Mgmt.	Chocolate weight management bar (Shaklee Corporation Pleasanton CA USA)	29	20	6			
B82	Meal Repl. & Weight Mgmt.	Cinch™ Café Latte weight management powder prepared with skim milk (Shaklee Corporation Pleasanton USA)	27	20	5			
B83	Meal Repl. & Weight Mgmt.	Cinch™ Chocolate weight management powder prepared with skim milk (Shaklee Corp.) USA)	16	20	3			
B84	Meal Repl. & Weight Mgmt.	Cinch™ Vanilla weight management powder prepared with skim milk	22	20	4			
C1330	Meal Repl. & Weight Mgmt.	Formula 1 Healthy Meal Nutritional Shake Mix: Caramel Apple (Herbalife International of America, Inc.) USA 2018*	15±2	20	3			
C1332	Meal Repl. & Weight Mgmt.	Formula 1 Healthy Meal Nutritional Shake Mix: Cookies and Cream (1 serve) + Protein Drink	29±4	20	6			

72

GLYCEMIC LOAD CARB COUNTER

Pub Ref f#	ISO Category	Food & Food Details	GI	ISO Avail Carb	ISO GL	Your Serv Size	Your Avail Carb	Your GL
		Mix: Vanilla (1/2 serve) + Prolessa Duo (1 serve) (Herbalife International of America, Inc.) USA 2019*						
C1333	Meal Repl. & Weight Mgmt.	Formula 1 Healthy Meal Nutritional Shake Mix: Cookies and Cream (1 serve) + Protein Drink Mix: Vanilla (1 serve) + Prolessa Duo (1 serve) (Herbalife International of America, Inc.) USA 2019*	29±4	20	6			
C1335	Meal Repl. & Weight Mgmt.	Formula 1 Healthy Meal Nutritional Shake Mix: French Vanilla (1 serve) + Protein Drink Mix: Vanilla (1 serve) + Prolessa Duo (1 serve) (Herbalife International of America, Inc.) USA 2019*	29±3	20	6			
C1334	Meal Repl. & Weight Mgmt.	Formula 1 Healthy Meal Nutritional Shake Mix: French Vanilla (1 serve) + Protein Drink Mix: Vanilla (1/2 serve) + Prolessa Duo (1 serve) (Herbalife	32±4	20	6			

GLYCEMIC LOAD CARB COUNTER

Pub Ref f#	ISO Category	Food & Food Details	GI	ISO Avail Carb	ISO GL	Your Serv Size	Your Avail Carb	Your GL
		International of America, Inc.) USA 2019*						
C1331	Meal Repl. & Weight Mgmt.	Formula 1 Healthy Meal Nutritional Shake Mix: Pralines & Cream (Herbalife International of America, Inc.) USA 2018*	15±2	20	3			
C1380	Meal repl. & Weight Mgmt.	Glucerna, diabetes-specific enteral formula (Abbott Laboratories Inc, USA)	15±3	20	3			
A476	Meal Repl. & Weight Mgmt.	L.E.A.N (Life long) Nutribar, peanut crunch	30	20	6			
A476	Meal Repl. & Weight Mgmt.	L.E.A.N Fibergy bar, harvest oat	45	20	9			
B1145	Meal Repl. & Weight Mgmt.	Lemon weight management bar (Shaklee Corporation USA)	23	20	5			
A54	Meal Repl. & Weight Mgmt.	Nutrimeal™ meal replacement drink Dutch Chocolate (Usana, Salt Lake City, USA)	26	20	5			
A476	Meal Repl. & Weight Mgmt.	Nutrimeal™ drink powder, Dutch chocolate	26	20	5			
C1353	Meal repl. & Weight Mgmt.	Nutrimeal™ Free Vanilla vegan meal replacement beverage	49±4	20	10			

Pub Ref f#	ISO Category	Food & Food Details	GI	ISO Avail Carb	ISO GL	Your Serv Size	Your Avail Carb	Your GL
		powder, prepared with 434.5 mL water (Usana Australia Pty Ltd, Baulkham Hills, Australia) USA 2013*						
B1148	Meal Repl. & Weight Mgmt.	Peanut Butter weight management bar (Shaklee Corporation, USA)	22	20	4			
C1398	Meal Repl. & Weight Mgmt.	Peptide 1.5 Plain nutrition formula (Kate Farms, Inc.) USA 2019*	26±4	20	5			
C1407	Meal Repl. & Weight Mgmt.	SDC (SDS (SUSTRA™ 2434 slowly digestible carbohydrate; blend of tapioca flour and corn starch) (Ingredion Incorporated, Bridgewater, NJ), prepared with water USA 2019*	27±2	20	5			
B1156	Meal Repl. & Weight Mgmt.	Slim Fast™ French Vanilla ready-to-drink shake (Slim Fast Foods Company Englewood USA)	37	20	7			
A476	Meal Repl. & Weight Mgmt.	Usana L.E.A.N (Life long) Nutribar™ Chocolate Crunch (Usana Inc, Salt Lake City, UT, US)	32	20	6			
A476	Meal Repl. &	Usana L.E.A.N (Life long)	30	20	6			

Pub Ref f#	ISO Category	Food & Food Details	GI	ISO Avail Carb	ISO GL	Your Serv Size	Your Avail Carb	Your GL
	Weight Mgmt.	Nutribar™ Peanut Crunch (Usana Inc, Salt Lake City, UT, US)						
A476	Meal Repl. & Weight Mgmt.	Usana L.E.A.N Fibergy™ bar Harvest Oat (Usana Inc, Salt Lake City, UT, US)	45	20	9			
A54	Meal Repl. & Weight Mgmt.	Usana Nutrimeal™ meal replacement drink powder Dutch Chocolate (Usana Inc, Salt Lake City, UT, US)	26	20	5			

NUTRITIONAL SUPPORT PDTS ISO 30g AVAIL CARB

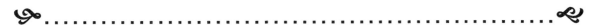

Pub Ref#	ISO Category	Food & Food Details	GI	ISO Avail Carb	ISO GL	Your Serv Size	Your Avail Carb	Your GL
B1275	Nutritional Support	Choicedm™ vanilla (Mead Johnson Nutritionals Evansville USA)	23	30	7			
A502	Nutritional Support	Enercal Plus, made from powder (Wyeth-Ayerst International Inc, Madison, NJ, US)	61	30	18			
B1279	Nutritional Support	Enercal Plus™, made from powder (Wyeth-Ayerst International Inc Madison USA)	61	30	18			
A507	Nutritional Support	Ensure Pudding, old-fashioned vanilla (Abbott Laboratories Inc, Ashland, OH, USA)	36	30	11			
B1288	Nutritional Support	Glucerna diabetes-specific enteral formula (Abbott Laboratories Inc USA)	15	30	5			
B1294	Nutritional Support	Glucerna SR diabetes-specific enteral formula (Abbott Laboratories Inc. USA)	23	30	7			
A508	Nutritional Support	Glucerna™ vanilla (Abbott Laboratories Inc. USA)6)	31	30	9			

GLYCEMIC LOAD CARB COUNTER

Pub Ref#	ISO Category	Food & Food Details	GI	ISO Avail Carb	ISO GL	Your Serv Size	Your Avail Carb	Your GL
A476	Nutritional Support	L.E.A.N (Life long) Nutribar, chocolate crunch	32	30	10			
B1303	Nutritional Support	Promote with fiber™ nutritional supplement (Ross Nutrition USA)	49	30	15			
C1410	Nutritional Support	Standard 1.0 Chocolate nutrition formula (Kate Farms, Inc., USA) USA 2019*	31±3	30	9			
C1411	Nutritional Support	Standard 1.0 Vanilla nutrition formula (Kate Farms, Inc., USA) USA 2019*	26±2	30	8			
C1412	Nutritional Support	Standard 1.4 Plain nutrition formula (Kate Farms, Inc., USA) USA 2019*	51±5	30	15			
A518	Nutritional Support	Ultracal™ with fiber (Mead Johnson, USA)	40	30	12			

NUTS ISO 5g AVAIL CARB

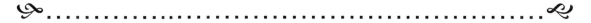

Pub Ref f#	ISO Category	Food & Food Details	GI	ISO Avail Carb	ISO GL	Your Serv Size	Your Avail Carb	Your GL
G	Nuts	Almonds	0	5	0			
G/H	Nuts	Cashews	25	5	1			
G	Nuts	Hazelnuts	0	5	0			
G	Nuts	Macadamia	0	5	0			
H	Nuts	Peanuts	7	5	0			
G	Nuts	Pecans	0	5	0			
G	Nuts	Walnuts	0	5	0			

PASTA ISO 40g AVAIL CARB

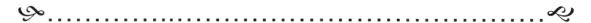

Pub Ref f#	ISO Category	Food & Food Details	GI	ISO Avail Carb	ISO GL	Your Serv Size	Your Avail Carb	Your GL
C1438b	Pasta	Barley pasta, cooked 5 min.; mean of five studies	62	40	25			
H	Pasta	Fettucine Pasta	32	40	13			
C1449b	Pasta	Gluten-free pasta, mean of nine foods 2015*	58	40	23			
C1491	Pasta	Low GI Noodles (Holista Biotech Corp., USA) USA 2017*	38±4	40	15			
H	Pasta	Macaroni and Cheese (Kraft®)	64	40	26			
H	Pasta	Macaroni, average	50	40	20			
B1351	Pasta	Proti pasta protein-enriched boiled in water (Vital Nature Inc San Antonio TX USA)	28	40	11			
C1502	Pasta	Rotini (Banza, LLC, USA) USA 2018*	44±9	40	18			
C1475b	Pasta	Spaghetti, white spaghetti, boiled, mean of 11 foods	47	40	19			
H	Pasta	Spaghetti, white, boiled 20 min.	58	40	23			
A534	Pasta	Spaghetti, white, Durum wheat, boiled 20 min (USA)	58	40	23			
A537	Pasta	Spaghetti, whole meal,	32	40	13			

GLYCEMIC LOAD CARB COUNTER

Pub Ref f#	ISO Category	Food & Food Details	GI	ISO Avail Carb	ISO GL	Your Serv Size	Your Avail Carb	Your GL
		boiled Whole meal (USA)						
H	Pasta	Spaghetti, whole-grain, boiled	42	40	17			
C1482b	Pasta	Wholemeal spaghetti, boiled for 8 min mean of five foods 2012*	50	40	20			

SNACKS & CONFECTIONERY ISO 25g AVAIL CARB

Pub Ref f#	ISO Category	Food & Food Details	GI	ISO Avail Carb	ISO GL	Your Serv Size	Your Avail Carb	Your GL
G	Snack/Confection	Apple slices with peanut butter	38	25	10			
G	Snack/Confection	Celery with Cashew Butter	40	25	10			
G	Snack/Confection	Celery with Hummus	40	25	10			
C1555b	Snack/Confection	Cheese Puffs, mean of four studies 2009*	63	25	16			
C1555	Snack/Confection	Cheese Puffs, Pirates Booty brand (Robert's American Gourmet, Sea Cliff, NY, USA), tested with coffee or tea USA 2009*	53±6	25	13			
C1602	Snack/Confection	Chocolate candy, sugar free, Dove® (M&M/Mars, USA) USA	23±3	25	6			
C1684	Snack/Sport Energy Bar	Chocolate Cherry Almond bar (Beachbody, LLC, USA) USA 2019*	22±2	25	6			
B1392	Snack/Confection	Chocolate dark Dove® (M&M/Mars USA)	23	25	6			
C1590b	Snack/Confection	Chocolate dark, mean of four foods	29	25	7			
C1595b	Snack/Confection	Chocolate, milk, plain, mean of four studies	45	25	11			
C1601b	Snack/Confection	Chocolate, white, mean of four studies	41	25	10			
B1503	Snack/Sport Energy Bar	Clif bar Chocolate Brownie Energy bar (Clif Bar Inc. Berkeley USA)	57	25	10			

GLYCEMIC LOAD CARB COUNTER

Pub Ref f#	ISO Category	Food & Food Details	GI	ISO Avail Carb	ISO GL	Your Serv Size	Your Avail Carb	Your GL
C1685	Snack/ Sport Energy Bar	Clif bar, Chocolate Brownie Energy bar (Clif Bar Inc., Berkeley, USA) USA	57±6	25	14			
B1471	Snack/Confection	Cocoavia™ Chocolate Almond Snack bar (M&M/Mars USA)	63	25	16			
B1472	Snack/ Confection	Cocoavia™ Cripsy Chocolate Bar (M&M/Mars USA)	33	25	8			
C1603	Snack/ Confection	Cocoavia™ high flavanol chocolate covered almonds (M&M/Mars, USA) USA	21±3	25	5			
C1603	Snack/ Confection	Cocoavia™ high flavanol chocolate covered almonds (M&M/Mars, USA) USA	21±3	25	5			
C1637	Snack/ Confection	Cold-pressed bar, made with 22.1 g maltodextrin (Globe Plus 10 DE maltodextrin) and 21.8 g corn syrup (Globe Plus 63 DE Maltodextrin) USA 2017*	93±8	25	23			
C1638	Snack/ Confection	Cold-pressed bar, made with 24.9 g SDS (SUSTRA™ 2434 slowly digestible carbohydrate) (Ingredion Incorporated, Bridgewater, NJ) and 18.9 g corn syrup (Globe Plus 63 DE Maltodextrin) USA 2017*	50±5	25	13			
B1401	Snack/ Confection	Combos Snacks Cheddar Cheese	54	25	14			

GLYCEMIC LOAD CARB COUNTER

Pub Ref f#	ISO Category	Food & Food Details	GI	ISO Avail Carb	ISO GL	Your Serv Size	Your Avail Carb	Your GL
		Crackers (M&M/Mars USA)						
C1550	Snack/ Confection	Combos Snacks Cheddar Cheese Crackers (M&M/Mars, USA)	54±6	25	14			
B1402	Snack/ Confection	Combos Snacks Cheddar Cheese Pretzels (M&M/Mars USA)	52	25	13			
H	Snack/ Confection	Corn chips	42	25	11			
G	Snack/ Confection	Dill Pickles	40	1*	<1			
G	Snack/ Confection	Egg, hardboiled	0	1*	0			
B1473	Snack/ Confection	ExtendBar™ Apple Cinnamon Delight Bar (ExtendBar USA)	33	25	8			
B1474	Snack/ Confection	ExtendBar™ Chocolate Delight Bar (ExtendBar USA)	41	25	10			
B1475	Snack/ Confection	ExtendBar™ Peanut Delight Bar (ExtendBar USA)	32	25	8			
H	Snack/ Confection	Fruit roll-Ups®	99	25	25			
H	Snack/ Confection	Graham crackers	74	25	19			
C1343	Snack/ Confection	Herbalife24 Achieve Protein Bar: Chocolate Chip Cookie Dough (Herbalife International of America, Inc.) USA 2017*	42±6	25	11			
C1342	Snack/ Confection	Herbalife24 Achieve Protein Bar: Dark Chocolate Brownie	49±8	25	12			

GLYCEMIC LOAD CARB COUNTER

Pub Ref f#	ISO Category	Food & Food Details	GI	ISO Avail Carb	ISO GL	Your Serv Size	Your Avail Carb	Your GL
		(Herbalife International of America, Inc.) USA 2017*						
H	Snack/ Confection	Hummus (chickpea salad dip), commercially prepared	6	25	2			
C1288	Snack/ Confection	Hummus (Sabra Classic Hummus; Sabra Dipping Co., S. Chesterfield, VA) USA 2016*	15± 3	25	4			
A570	Snack/ Sport Energy Bar	Ironman PR bar, chocolate (PR Nutrition, San Diego, CA, USA)	39	25	10			
B1507	Snack/ Sport Energy Bar	Ironman PR bar® chocolate (PR Nutrition San Diego CA USA)	39	25	10			
C1656	Snack/ Confection	KitKat (Nestlè, Italy) Italy 2012*	50± 7	25	13			
B1434	Snack/ Confection	Kudos Milk Chocolate Granola bar with M&M's Milk Chocolate Mini Baking Bits (M&M/Mars USA)	52	25	13			
B1436	Snack/ Confection	Kudos Milk Chocolate Granola bars Peanut Butter flavor (M&M/Mars USA)	45	25	11			
B1435	Snack/ Confection	Kudos Whole-Grain bars chocolate chip (M&M/Mars Hackettstown USA)	62	25	16			
A551	Snack/ Confection	Kudos Whole-Grain Bars, chocolate chip (M & M/Mars, Hackettstown, NJ, USA)	62	25	16			

GLYCEMIC LOAD CARB COUNTER

Pub Ref f#	ISO Category	Food & Food Details	GI	ISO Avail Carb	ISO GL	Your Serv Size	Your Avail Carb	Your GL
C1610	Snack/ Confection	Licorice pieces Australia 2012*	69±8	25	17			
H	Snack/ Confection	M&M's®, peanut	33	25	8			
A554	Snack/ Confection	Mars Bar Mars Bar (M & M/Mars, USA)	68	25	17			
B1441	Snack/ Confection	Mars Bar® (M&M/Mars USA)	68	25	17			
C1616	Snack/ Confection	Marshmallows (Woolworths Homebrand, Australia) Australia 2012*	67±4	25	17			
B1443	Snack/ Confection	Milky Way® bar (M&M/Mars USA)	62	25	16			
C1660	Snack/ Confection	Milky Way® bar (M&M/Mars, USA) USA 1997	62±8	25	16			
B1444	Snack/ Confection	Milky Way® Lite bar (M&M/Mars USA)	45	25	11			
C1661	Snack/ Confection	Milky Way® Lite bar (M&M/Mars, USA) USA 1997	45±5	25	11			
B1477	Snack/ Confection	Munch Peanut Butter bar (M&M/Mars USA)	27	25	7			
C1662	Snack/ Confection	Munch Peanut Butter bar (M&M/Mars, USA) USA 2004	27±5	25	7			
C1620b	Snack/ Confection	Nutella® (Ferrero, Italy) Italy 2012*, mean of four studies	33	25	8			
1663	Snacks/ Confection	Nuts and Seeds Superfoods bar (SoLo GI Nutrition, Inc, Canada) Canada 2018*	33±6	25	8			
C1688	Snack/ Confection	Peanut Butter Chocolate bar (Beachbody, LLC) USA 2019*	32±4	25	8			

GLYCEMIC LOAD CARB COUNTER

Pub Ref f#	ISO Category	Food & Food Details	GI	ISO Avail Carb	ISO GL	Your Serv Size	Your Avail Carb	Your GL
C1688	Snack/ Sport Energy Bar	Peanut Butter Chocolate bar (Beachbody, LLC) USA 2019*	32± 4	25	8			
C1667	Snack/ Confection	Peanut Butter Chocolate Pal™ bar (Revival Soy®, Physicians Pharmaceuticals, Inc., USA) USA	52± 4	25	13			
C1689	Snack/ Sport Energy Bar	Performance Chocolate Energy bar (Power Bar, USA)	53± 6	25	13			
B1504	Snack/ Sport Energy Bar	Performance Chocolate Energy bar (Power Bar USA) Power Bar® (Powerfood Inc. Berkeley USA)	53	25	13			
B1450	Snack/ Confection	Pirate's Booty aged white cheddar extruded snack made from corn and rice (Robert's American Gourmet Sea Cliff NY USA)	70	25	18			
C68	Snack/ Confection	Pizza base, baked in oven at 220°C for 9 min (Boboli, Orograin Bakeries Manufacturing Inc, PA, USA) USA 2015*	52± 4	25	13			
H	Snack/ Confection	Pizza, plain baked dough, served with parmesan cheese and tomato sauce	80	25	20			
H	Snack/ Confection	Pizza, Super Supreme (Pizza Hut®)	36	25	9			
H	Snack/ Confection	Popcorn, Microwave popcorn plain, average	55	25	14			

Pub Ref f#	ISO Category	Food & Food Details	GI	ISO Avail Carb	ISO GL	Your Serv Size	Your Avail Carb	Your GL
C1572b	Snack/Confection	Popcorn, microwave popcorn mean of 5 studies	62	25	16			
C1568	Snack/Confection	Poppin Microwave Popcorn, butter flavor (Green's Foods, Australia) Australia 2013*	51±6	25	13			
H	Snack/Confection	Potato chips, average	56	25	14			
C1573	Snack/Confection	Potato chips, crinkle cut, Smith's™ Original Australia 2012*	48±5	25	12			
C1574	Snack/Confection	Potato chips, Pringles™ Original Australia 2012*	57±5	25	14			
C1578		Potato chips, Sweet potato crisps, Red Rock Deli™ (The Red Rock Deli Chip Company, VIC, Australia) Australia 2016*	41±4	25	10			
C1577b	Snack/Confection	Potato crisps, mean of five studies 56	56	25	14			
C1690	Snack/ Sport Energy Bar	Power Bar®, chocolate (Powerfood Inc., Berkeley, USA)	58±5	25	15			
C207	Snack/Confection	Pretzel, Soft pretzel, soy USA 2011*	39±6	25	10			
C208	Snack/Confection	Pretzel, Soft pretzel, wheat USA 2011*	66±4	25	17			
H	Snack/Confection	Pretzels, oven-baked	83	25	21			
USDA/JL	Snack/Confection	Ranger Cookies, 2, (Flourless) (From recipe in *Are You Sweet Enough Already?*)	35	9*	3			

GLYCEMIC LOAD CARB COUNTER

Pub Ref f#	ISO Category	Food & Food Details	GI	ISO Avail Carb	ISO GL	Your Serv Size	Your Avail Carb	Your GL
H	Snack/ Confection	Rice cakes, average	82	25	21			
B731	Snack/ Confection	Rice, Puffed rice cakes caramel flavored (USA)	82	25	21			
H	Snack/ Confection	Rye crisps, average	64	25	16			
G	Snack/ Confection	Sardines, fish snacks, canned	0	0*	0			
H	Snack/ Confection	Shortbread	64	25	16			
C1629	Snack/ Confection	Skittles® (Mars Confectionery, Australia) Australia	70±5	25	18			
B1481	Snack/ Confection	Slimfast™ Meal Options bar rich chocolate brownie (SlimFast Foods Co West Palm Beach USA)	64	25	16			
C1691	Snack/ Sport Energy Bar	SmartZone Chocolate flavor, Nutrition bar (Hershey's Food Corporation, Hershey, PA, USA)	16±3	25	4			
C1692	Snack/ Sport Energy Bar	SmartZone Crunchy Blueberry flavor, Nutrition bar (Hershey's Food Corporation, Hershey, PA, USA)	15±3	25	4			
C1693	Snack/ Sport Energy Bar	SmartZone Crunchy Chocolate Brownie flavor, Nutrition bar (Hershey's Food Corporation, Hershey, PA, USA)	23±5	25	6			
C1694	Snack/	SmartZone Crunchy	16±4	25	4			

GLYCEMIC LOAD CARB COUNTER

Pub Ref f#	ISO Category	Food & Food Details	GI	ISO Avail Carb	ISO GL	Your Serv Size	Your Avail Carb	Your GL
	Sport Energy Bar	Chocolate Caramel flavor, Nutrition bar (Hershey's Food Corporation, Hershey, PA, USA)						
C1695	Snack/ Sport Energy Bar	SmartZone Crunchy Chocolate Peanut Butter flavor, Nutrition bar (Hershey's Food Corporation, Hershey, PA, USA)	14±3	25	4			
C1696	Snack/ Sport Energy Bar	SmartZone Crunchy Key Lime flavor, Nutrition bar (Hershey's Food Corporation, Hershey, PA, USA)	14±3	25	4			
B1509	Snack/ Sport Energy Bar	SmartZone Nutrition Bar Chocolate flavor (Hershey Foods Corp. Hershey PA, USA.)	16	25	4			
B1510	Snack/ Sport Energy Bar	SmartZone Nutrition Bar Crunchy Blueberry flavor	15	25	4			
B1511	Snack/ Sport Energy Bar	SmartZone Nutrition Bar Crunchy Chocolate Brownie flavor	23	25	6			
B1512	Snack/ Sport Energy Bar	SmartZone Nutrition Bar Crunchy Chocolate Caramel flavor	16	25	4			
B1513	Snack/ Sport Energy Bar	SmartZone Nutrition Bar Crunchy	14	25	4			

GLYCEMIC LOAD CARB COUNTER

Pub Ref f#	ISO Category	Food & Food Details	GI	ISO Avail Carb	ISO GL	Your Serv Size	Your Avail Carb	Your GL
		Chocolate Peanut Butter flavor						
B1514	Snack/ Sport Energy Bar	SmartZone Nutrition Bar Crunchy Key Lime flavor	14	25	4			
B1515	Snack/ Sport Energy Bar	SmartZone Nutrition Bar Peanut Butter flavor	18	25	5			
		Snickers® Marathon Energy Bar (Hershey's Food Corporation, Hershey PA,USA)						
B1508	Snack/ Sport Energy Bar	SmartZone Nutrition Bar Chocolate flavor	11	25	3			
C1697	Snack/ Sport Energy Bar	SmartZone Peanut Butter flavor, Nutrition bar (Hershey's Food Corporation, Hershey, PA, USA)	18± 2	25	5			
B1482	Snack/ Confection	Snack bar Apple Cinnamon (Con Agra Inc. Omaha NE USA)	40	25	10			
B1483	Snack/ Confection	Snack bar Peanut Butter and Choc-Chip (Con Agra Inc. USA)	37	25	9			
A565	Snack/ Confection	Snack bar, apple cinnamon (Con Agra Inc, USA)	40	25	10			
A565	Snack/ Confection	Snack bar, peanut butter and choc-chip (Con Agra Inc, USA)	37	25	9			
A566	Snack/ Confection	Snickers Bar® (M & M/Mars, USA)	68	25	17			
B1487	Snack/ Confection	Snickers Bar® (M&M/Mars USA)	43	25	11			
H	Snack/ Confection	Snickers Bar®, average	51	25	13			

GLYCEMIC LOAD CARB COUNTER

Pub Ref f#	ISO Category	Food & Food Details	GI	ISO Avail Carb	ISO GL	Your Serv Size	Your Avail Carb	Your GL
B1517	Snack/ Sport Energy Bar	Snickers® (M&M/Mars, USA) Marathon Energy Bar Cookies & Crème flavor	50	25	13			
B1522	Snack/ Sport Energy Bar	Snickers® (M&M/Mars, USA) Marathon Nutrition Bar Dark Chocolate Crunch flavor	49	25	12			
B1518	Snack/ Sport Energy Bar	Snickers® Marathon Energy Bar Multi Grain Crunch flavor	50	25	13			
B1519	Snack/ Sport Energy Bar	Snickers® Marathon Energy Bar Peanut Butter flavor	34	25	9			
B1516	Snack/ Sport Energy Bar	Snickers® Marathon Energy Bar Chewy Chocolate Peanut flavor	36	25	9			
C1698	Snack/ Sport Energy Bar	Snickers® Marathon Energy bar, Chewy Chocolate Peanut flavor (M&M/Mars, USA)	36±5	25	9			
C1699	Snack/ Sport Energy Bar	Snickers® Marathon Energy bar, Cookies & Crème flavor (M&M/Mars, USA)	50±4	25	13			
C1700	Snack/ Sport Energy Bar	Snickers® Marathon Energy bar, Multi Grain Crunch flavor (M&M/Mars, USA)	50±4	25	13			
C1701	Snack/ Sport Energy Bar	Snickers® Marathon Energy bar, Peanut Butter flavor (M&M/Mars, USA)	34±5	25	9			
C1702	Snack/	Snickers® Marathon Low	20±4	25	5			

GLYCEMIC LOAD CARB COUNTER

Pub Ref f#	ISO Category	Food & Food Details	GI	ISO Avail Carb	ISO GL	Your Serv Size	Your Avail Carb	Your GL
	Sport Energy Bar	Carb Lifestyle Energy bar, Chocolate Fudge Brownie flavor (M&M/Mars, USA)						
C1703	Snack/ Sport Energy Bar	Snickers® Marathon Low Carb Lifestyle Energy bar, Peanut Butter flavor (M&M/Mars, USA)	21±4	25	5			
B1521	Snack/ Sport Energy Bar	Snickers® Marathon Low Carb Lifestyle Energy Bar Peanut Butter flavor	21	25	5			
B1520	Snack/ Sport Energy Bar	Snickers® Marathon Low Carb Lifestyle Energy Bar Chocolate Fudge Brownie flavor	20	25	5			
C1704	Snack/ Sport Energy Bar	Snickers® Marathon Nutrition bar, Dark Chocolate Crunch flavor (M&M/Mars, USA)	49±6	25	12			
C1705	Snack/ Sport Energy Bar	Snickers® Marathon Nutrition bar, Honey & Roasted Almond flavor (M&M/Mars, USA)	41±3	25	10			
B1523	Snack/ Sport Energy Bar	Snickers® Marathon Nutrition Bar Honey & Roasted Almond flavor	41	25	10			
C1706	Snack/ Sport Energy Bar	Snickers® Marathon Protein Performance bar, Caramel Nut	26±3	25	7			

GLYCEMIC LOAD CARB COUNTER

Pub Ref f#	ISO Category	Food & Food Details	GI	ISO Avail Carb	ISO GL	Your Serv Size	Your Avail Carb	Your GL
		Rush flavor (M&M/Mars, USA)						
C1707	Snack/ Sport Energy Bar	Snickers® Marathon Protein Performance bar, Chocolate Nut Burst flavor (M&M/Mars, USA)	32±4	25	8			
B1524	Snack/ Sport Energy Bar	Snickers® Marathon Protein Performance Bar (M&M/Mars, USA) Caramel Nut Rush flavor	26	25	7			
B1525	Snack/ Sport Energy Bar	Snickers® Marathon Protein Performance Bar Chocolate Nut Burst flavor	32	25	8			
C1582	Snack/ Confection	Soy chips, Sunshine™ soy protein chips, lightly salted (Revival Soy®, Physicians Pharmaceuticals, Inc., USA) USA 2004	87±8	25	22			
B1425	Snack/ Confection	Strawberry fruit leather (Stretch Island Fruit Company™ Washington USA)	25	25	6			
C1544b	Snack/ Confection	Strawberry Fruit Leather, mean of 3 foods	27	25	7			
C1542	Snack/ Confection	Sweet strawberry fruit leather (Stretch Island Fruit Company™, WA, USA), tested with water USA 2009*	25±5	25	6			
C1543	Snack/ Confection	Sweet strawberry fruit leather	22±3	25	6			

GLYCEMIC LOAD CARB COUNTER

Pub Ref f#	ISO Category	Food & Food Details	GI	ISO Avail Carb	ISO GL	Your Serv Size	Your Avail Carb	Your GL
		(Stretch Island Fruit Company™, WA, USA), tested with coffee or tea USA 2009*						
C1544	Snack/ Confection	Sweet strawberry fruit leather (Stretch Island Fruit Co, Allyn, WA, USA) USA 2008*	33±7	25	8			
C1683	Snack/ Sport Energy Bar	Twix® Cookie Bar, caramel (M&M/Mars, USA) USA	44±6	25	11			
B1536	Snack/ Sport Energy Bar	VO2 Max Chocolate Energy bar (M&M/Mars USA)	49	25	12			
C1718	Snack/ Sport Energy Bar	VO2 Max Chocolate Energy bar (M&M/Mars, USA)	49±8	25	12			
B1537	Snack/ Sport Energy Bar	ZonePerfect Nutrition bar Double Chocolate flavor (Abbott Laboratories Abbott Park USA)	44	25	11			

SOUP ISO 20g AVAIL CARB

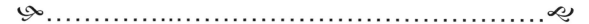

Pub Ref f#	ISO Category	Food & Food Details	GI	ISO Avail Carb	ISO GL	Your Serv Size	Your Avail Carb	Your GL
A571	Soup	Black Bean Soup (Wil-Pack Foods, San Pedro, CA, USA)	64	20	13			
C1724	Soup	Chunky Roast Chicken and Vegetable soup (Campbell's Soups, Homebush, NSW, Australia) Australia 2016*	52±3	20	10			
B1546/C1727	Soup	Minestrone condensed soup prepared with water (Campbell's Soup Company Camden NJ USA)	48	20	10			
C1732	Soup	Potato & Bacon soup, chunky (Campbell's Soups, Homebush, NSW, Australia) Australia 2016*	41±4	20	8			
A576	Soup	Split Pea Soup (Wil-Pak Foods, USA)	60	20	12			
B1555/C1735	Soup	Tomato soup condensed prepared with water (Campbell's Soup Company Camden NJ USA)	52	20	10			

SUGARS & SYRUPS ISO 5g AVAIL CARB

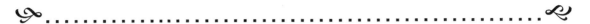

Pub Ref #	ISO Category	Food & Food Details	GI	ISO Avail Carb	ISO GL	Your Serv Size	Your Avail Carb	Your GL
B1563	Sweetener	Agave honey, Premium Agave nectar (Sweet Cactus Farms USA), mean of three studies	19	5	1			
C1740	Sweetener	Agave, Organic Cactus Nectar, light, 90% fructose (Western Commerce Corp., City of Industry, CA, USA)	11±1	5	1			
C1741	Sweetener	Agave, Organic Cactus Nectar, light, 97% fructose (Western Commerce Corp., USA)	10±1	5	1			
C1742	Sweetener	Agave, Premium nectar (Sweet Cactus Farms, USA) USA	19±4	5	1			
G	Sweetener	Blackstrap molasses	55	5	3			
B1593	Sweetener	Buckwheat honey ratio of fructose: glucose 1.12 (Vazza Farms USA)	73	5	4			
C1761	Sweetener	Buckwheat honey, ratio of fructose:glucose, 1.12 Vazza Farms, USA) USA	73±6	5	4			
B1591	Sweetener	Clover honey ratio of fructose:	69	5	3			

GLYCEMIC LOAD CARB COUNTER

Pub Ref #	ISO Category	Food & Food Details	GI	ISO Avail Carb	ISO GL	Your Serv Size	Your Avail Carb	Your GL
		glucose 1.09 (Vazza Farms Hermiston OR USA)						
C1759	Sweetener	Clover honey, ratio of fructose: glucose, 1.09 (Vazza Farms, Hermiston, OR, USA)	69±8	5	3			
C1779	Sweetener	Coconut sugar, organic, Loving Earth™ brand Indonesia 2014*	54±6	5	3			
C1762	Sweetener	Cotton honey, ratio of fructose:glucose, 1.03 (Gene Brandi Apiaries, Los Banos, CA, USA)	74±7	5	4			
C1780	Sweetener	Dates Syrup, Gurun Emas (Omni Mal Agencies Sdn. Bhd, Malaysia) Malaysia 2018*	54±4	5	3			
C1128b	Sweetener	Dates, mean of 19 foods	54	5	3			
A580	Sweetener	Fructose, 50g. (Sigma Chemical Co., St. Louis, MO, USA)	24	5	1			
C1744b	Sweetener	Fructose, mean of two studies 24	24	5	1			
C1747	Sweetener	Glucose syrup Australia 2014*	107±7	5	5			
C1745	Sweetener	High fructose corn syrup Australia 2014*	56±5	5	3			
C1476	Sweetener	High fructose corn syrup with 3.3 g Filtered Molasses	50±3	5	3			

GLYCEMIC LOAD CARB COUNTER

Pub Ref #	ISO Category	Food & Food Details	GI	ISO Avail Carb	ISO GL	Your Serv Size	Your Avail Carb	Your GL
		Concentrate added per 100 g (4.16 g FMC/100 g carbohydrate) Australia 2014*						
C1764b	Sweetener	Honey, mean of 17 types of honey	60	5	3			
C1783	Sweetener	Karo Dark Corn Syrup USA 2013*	90±6	5	5			
A587	Sweetener	Lactose, 50g. (Sigma Chemical Co., USA	43	5	2			
C1767b	Sweetener	Maltose, mean of two studies	90	5	5			
C1758	Sweetener	Manuka honey, MGO 440+ (Manuka Health New Zealand Ltd) New Zealand 2011*	65±7	5	3			
C1785	Sweetener	Maple syrup, pure Canadian (Queen Foods, Australia) Canada	54±6	5	3			
C1786	Sweetener	Rice malt syrup (Pure Harvest Organic, Australia) Australia 2013*	98±6	5	5			
Pkg	Sweetener	Stevia powder	0	1*	0			
Pkg	Sweetener	Stevia extract	0	0*	0			
C1776	Sweetener	Sucrose (LoGiCane) (Horizon Science, Australia)13 Australia 2014*	62±4	5	3			
A589	Sweetener	Sucrose, 50g. (Sigma Chemical Co. USA)	58	5	3			

Pub Ref #	ISO Category	Food & Food Details	GI	ISO Avail Carb	ISO GL	Your Serv Size	Your Avail Carb	Your GL
C1769	Sweetener	Sucrose, cane sugar Australia 2016*	60±4	5	3			
C1774b	Sweetener	Sucrose, mean of 7 studies	66					
C1787	Sweetener	Sugar, from organic fruits (Dolcedì, zucchero da frutta biologica, Rigoni di Asiago, Italy) Italy 2009*	23±5	5	1			
C1777	Sweetener	Sugar, refined (Sadam-Eridania, Italy) Italy 2013*	91±10	5	5			
B1596	Sweetener	Tupelo honey ratio of fructose: glucose 1.54 (Tropical Blossom Honey Co Edgewater FL USA)	74	5	4			
C1764	Sweetener	Tupelo honey, ratio of fructose:glucose, 1.54 (Tropical Blossom Honey Co, Edgewater, FL, USA) USA	74±8	5	4			
G	Sweetener	Xylitol 2.5g	7	2.5*	0.2			

VEGETABLES ISO 20g AVAIL CARB

Pub Ref #	ISO Category	Food & Food Details	ISO GI	ISO Avail Carb	ISO GL	Your Serv Size	Your Avail Carb	Your GL
G	Vegetable	Artichoke	40	20	8			
G	Vegetable	Arugula	40	20	8			
G	Vegetable	Asparagus	40	20	8			
G	Vegetable	Beet greens	40	20	8			
G	Vegetable	Beet root	40	10*	4*			
G	Vegetable	Bell pepper	40	20	8			
G	Vegetable	Bok Choy	40	20	8			
G	Vegetable	Broccoli	40	20	8			
G	Vegetable	Cabbage	40	20	8			
H	Vegetable	Carrots, average	39	10*	4*			
C1805	Vegetable	Carrots, diced, frozen (Talleys Group Ltd) 13 New Zealand 2011*	31±2	10*	3*			
C1804	Vegetable	Carrots, unpeeled, boiled Australia 2020*	32±4	10*	3*			
G	Vegetable	Cauliflower	40	20	8			
G	Vegetable	Celery	40	20	8			
G	Vegetable	Collard greens	40	20	8			
C1801	Vegetable	Corn, Sweet corn, cooked in microwave for 1.5 min Australia 2015*	51±4	20	10			
G	Vegetable	Cucumber	40	20	8			
G	Vegetable	Dandelion greens	40	20	8			
G	Vegetable	Eggplant	40	20	8			
G	Vegetable	Garlic	40	20	8			
G	Vegetable	Ginger root	40	20	5			
G	Vegetable	Grape leaves	40	20	8			
G	Vegetable	Green beans	40	20	8			
G	Vegetable	Green Leaf Lettuce	0	4*	0			
H	Vegetable	Green peas, average	54	10*	5*			

GLYCEMIC LOAD CARB COUNTER

Pub Ref #	ISO Category	Food & Food Details	ISO GI	ISO Avail Carb	ISO GL	Your Serv Size	Your Avail Carb	Your GL
C1798		Green Peas, frozen, heated in the microwave (McCain Foods Aust. Pty Ltd, Australia) Australia 2020*	42±4	10*	4			
C1797	Vegetable	Green Peas, plain and frozen (Talleys Group Ltd, New Zealand)13 New Zealand 2011*	29±2	10*	3			
C1860b	Vegetable	Instant mashed potato, mean of five studies	84	20	17			
G	Vegetable	Jicama	40	20	8			
G	Vegetable	Kale	40	20	8			
G	Vegetable	Kohlrabi	40	20	8			
G	Vegetable	Leek	40	20	8			
G	Vegetable	Mushrooms	40	20	8			
G	Vegetable	Mustard greens	40	20	8			
A747	Vegetable	Nopal (prickly pear cactus)	7	20	8			
G	Vegetable	Okra	40	20	8			
G	Vegetable	Olives	40	20	8			
G	Vegetable	Onion	40	20	8			
H	Vegetable	Parsnips	52	10*	5*			
C1852b	Vegetable	Potato cooked then cooled, mean of 8 foods	49	20	10			
B1631	Vegetable	Potato, baked russet	111	20	22			
C1838b	Vegetable	Potato, Boiled potato, mean of 29 foods	73	20	15			
C1870	Vegetable	Potato, California white	72±8	20	14			

102

GLYCEMIC LOAD CARB COUNTER

Pub Ref #	ISO Category	Food & Food Details	ISO GI	ISO Avail Carb	ISO GL	Your Serv Size	Your Avail Carb	Your GL
		potatoes, cubed, roasted in soybean oil USA						
B1658	Vegetable	Potato, French fries (Oreida Golden Fries)	64	20	13			
C1854	Vegetable	Potato, French Fries, baked 15 min (Oreida Golden Fries, H.J. Heinz Co, Pittsburgh, PA, USA)	64±6	20	13			
C1872	Vegetables	Potato, Hash Browns, crispy shredded potato cakes, frozen, baked at 230oC for 17 min, Birds Eye™ Australia 2012*	56±6	20	11			
B1660	Vegetable	Potato, instant mashed (Idahoan Foods)	79	20	16			
C1856	Vegetable	Potato, Instant mashed potato (Idahoan Foods, Lewisville, ID, USA) USA	88±8	20	18			
C1857	Vegetable	Potato, Instant mashed potato (Idahoan Foods, Lewisville, ID, USA), prepared with water USA	92±4	20	18			
C1858	Vegetable	Potato, Instant mashed potato (Idahoan Foods,	69±9	20	14			

GLYCEMIC LOAD CARB COUNTER

Pub Ref #	ISO Category	Food & Food Details	ISO GI	ISO Avail Carb	ISO GL	Your Serv Size	Your Avail Carb	Your GL
		Lewisville, ID, USA), prepared with water USA						
C1859	Vegetable	Potato, Instant mashed potato (Idahoan Foods, Lewisville, ID, USA) USA	97±6	20	19			
H	Vegetable	Potato, instant mashed, average	87	20	17			
C1865b	Vegetable	Potato, Mashed potato, mean of five studies	79	20	16			
C1898	Vegetable	Potato, Red sweet potato (Ipomoea batatas), NS, cooking method NS13 New Zealand 2011*	84±6	20	17			
B1655	Vegetable Potato Special Info.	Potato, red, cubed, boiled in salted water 12 min, stored overnight in refrigerator, consumed cold (Canada)	56	20	11			
C1869	Vegetable	Potato, Russet Burbank Norkotah potato, unpeeled, cooked in microwave for 18 min USA	77±9	20	15			
B1646	Vegetable Potato Special Info.	Potato, Sava, peeled, boiled 21-30 min (Sweden)	118	20	24			
B1653	Vegetable Potato	Potato, Sava, peeled, boiled	67	20	13			

GLYCEMIC LOAD CARB COUNTER

Pub Ref #	ISO Category	Food & Food Details	ISO GI	ISO Avail Carb	ISO GL	Your Serv Size	Your Avail Carb	Your GL
	Special Info.	21-30 min, refrigerated 24 h, consumed cold with white vinegar (28 g) and olive oil (8g) (Sweden)						
H	Vegetable	Potato, sweet potato, average	70	20	14			
C1884b	Vegetable	Potato, Sweet potato, baked with skin on for 45 min., mean of 11 studies	88	20	18			
C1910b	Vegetable	Potato, sweet potato, fried in preheated vegetable oil, mean of 11 studies	71	20	14			
C1921b	Vegetable	Potato, sweet potato, roasted over pre-heated charcoal for 45 min., mean of 11 studies	86	20	17			
B1654	Vegetable Potato Special Info.	Potato, Type NS, boiled in salted water, refrigerated, reheated (India)	23	20	8			
H	Vegetable	Potato, white, boiled, average	82	20	16			
H	Vegetable	Potato, yam, average	54	20	11			
B1665	Vegetable	Potatoes, Instant mashed potatoes (Idahoan Foods	97	20	19			

GLYCEMIC LOAD CARB COUNTER

Pub Ref #	ISO Category	Food & Food Details	ISO GI	ISO Avail Carb	ISO GL	Your Serv Size	Your Avail Carb	Your GL
		Lewisville ID USA)						
A603	Vegetable	Potatoes, Russet Burbank potatoes, baked without fat, 45-60 min (USA)	78	20	20			
A603	Vegetable	Potatoes, Russet, baked without fat (USA)	94	20	19			
A603	Vegetable	Potatoes, Russet, baked without fat (USA)	111	20	22			
C1799	Fruit	Pumpkin, Butternut pumpkin, boiled Australia 2006	51±6	10*	5*			
G	Vegetable	Radicchio	40	20	8			
G	Vegetable	Radish	40	20	8			
G	Vegetable	Spinach	0	4*	0			
B504	Grain	Sweet corn	60	20	12			
A265	Grain	Sweet corn (USA)	60	20	12			
H	Grain	Sweet corn on the cob	48	20	9			
B1619	Grain	Sweet corn, boiled	60	20	12			
A597	Grain	Sweet corn, whole-kernel, diet pack, Featherweight, canned, drained, heated, USA	46	20	12			
C1897b	Vegetable	Sweet Potato, boiled, mean of 13 studies	46	20	9			
G	Vegetable	Swiss chard	40	20	8			
G	Vegetable	Tomatillo	40	20	8			
G	Fruit	Tomato (Solanum	23	15*	3			

GLYCEMIC LOAD CARB COUNTER

Pub Ref #	ISO Category	Food & Food Details	ISO GI	ISO Avail Carb	ISO GL	Your Serv Size	Your Avail Carb	Your GL
		lycopersicum), raw						
C1946	Vegetable Product	Tomato and vegetable pasta sauce, commercially-prepared France 2007	23±3	10*	2*			
B1058	Fruit	Tomato juice, canned	38	10*	4			
C1202	Fruit	Tomato juice, canned, no added sugar (Berri Ltd, Australia) Australia 2002	38±4	10*	4			
C1945	Vegetable Product	Tomato sauce, with extra cheese (Pasta Bake, Dolmio, Mars Foods, New Zealand) New Zealand 2011*	35±3	10*	4			
G	Vegetable	Turmeric root	40	20	8			
G	Vegetable	Watercress	40	2*	1			
G	Vegetable	Wheatgrass	40	20	8			
C1941b	Vegetable	Yam, mean of 21 foods	68	20	14			
G	Vegetable	Zucchini	40	20	8			

TROUBLESHOOTING

FOOD & FOOD DETAILS	EXPERIENCE	DATE & TIME	GI	Your Serv Size	Your Avail Carbs	Your GL

GLYCEMIC LOAD CARB COUNTER

FOOD & FOOD DETAILS	EXPERIENCE	DATE & TIME	GI	Serv Size	Avail Carbs	GL

MEAL PREP NOTES

ENDNOTES, REFERENCES & RESOURSES

[i] In all of the tables of this book, the first column is "Pub Ref #." This is the "published reference number." This number refers to the source (A, B, C, etc., as listed below) and the test number of the information presented in the table. More than one reference is used in some cases. A "/" separates any multiple reference sources.

Here are the information resources used in the preparation of these tables:

- "A" = *International Tables of Glycemic Index and Glycemic Load Values, 2002.* The US National Library of Medicine, National Institutes of Health, archives this research. The individual tables of glycemic study results are available at: https://www.ncbi.nlm.nih.gov/pubmed/12081815 This table contains nearly 1,300 study results from countries all over the world. The location and exact study number of each test result is referenced in the tables of this book for your convenience.

- "B" = *International Tables of Glycemic Index and Glycemic Load Values, 2008.* Here is the entire article: https://www.ncbi.nlm.nih.gov/pmc/articles/PMC2584181/ This research is archived by the US National Library of Medicine, National Institutes of Health. The individual tables of glycemic study results are available at: https://www.ncbi.nlm.nih.gov/pmc/articles/PMC2584181/bin/dc08-1239_index.html. This table contain 2,478 of these individual food study results from countries all over the world. The location and exact study number of the each test is referenced in the tables of this book for your convenience.

"C" = *International Tables of Glycemic Index and Glycemic Load Values, 2021: A Systematic Review.* The tables included in this article provide International Standards Organization measuring system regarding Glycemic Load. Here is the link to the entire article: https://pubmed.ncbi.nlm.nih.gov/34258626/. This research is archived by the US National Library of Medicine, National Institutes of Health. These tables contain over 4,000 entries from countries all over the world. The location and exact study number of each test result is referenced in the tables of this book for your convenience.

- "G" = Glycemicindex.com. http://www.glycemicindex.com/

- "H" = Harvard University: http://www.health.harvard.edu/diseases-and-conditions/glycemic_index_and_glycaemic_load_for_100_foods

- "USDA" = USDA National Nutrient Database for Standard Reference is a listing of 8,789 foods. The United States Department of Agriculture database provides information for carbohydrate content in *GLYCEMIC LOAD MASTERY*. You can access the USDA Nutrient Database at Food Data Central here: https://fdc.nal.usda.gov/

- "PKG" = Portions of nutritional information is provided from the product packaging.

- "#" = Fruits lacking a lab-tested glycemic index test score are given a value based on a simple arithmetic calculation. A total of all tested fruits' GI scores were added together and divided by the total number of tested fruit scores. There are 22 fruits with lab-tested scores, the total of their scores adding up to 870. 870 divided by the 22 fruits = 39.55.

This was done to verify the accuracy of Glycemic Index "assignment." Assignment began when it was not humanly possible to consume 50g carbohydrate portions of many foods in order to conduct testing. Since a fruit is part of the vegetable family, and any untested vegetable is assigned a GI score of 40, any untested fruits are therefore assigned a GI value of 40.

- For other books by this author please see: amazon.com/author/judylickus

- Learn more details about carbohydrates, glycemic index, and glycemic load at the free informational blog: LowGlycemicHappiness.com

- Like the Low Glycemic Happiness Facebook page for news & updates at: Facebook.com/LowGlycemicHappiness

- Other Books by this Author:

For more on Glycemic Load please see *Glycemic Load Food Guide* at Amazon, booksellers, and libraries. This book emphasizes the science involved in establishing a low glycemic load lifestyle through food choice, serving, and preparation for a variety of medical conditions. It also includes an exclusive Glycemic Load Personal Workbook to help you track your scores.

For metric serving sizes of Carbs, GI, Fiber, and GL of USA foods, please see *Cheat Sheet Simply for USA Foods* available in paperback and EBook at Amazon, booksellers, and libraries.

For Canadian Glycemic Values (metric serving sizes) of Carbs, GI, Fiber, and GL of Canadian foods, please see *Cheat Sheet Simply for Canadian Foods* available in paperback and EBook at Amazon, booksellers, and libraries.

For Great Britain foods (metric serving sizes) of Carbs, GI, Fiber, and GL of UK foods, please see *Cheat Sheet Simply for UK Foods* available in paperback and EBook at Amazon, booksellers, and libraries.

Nutrient Essentials provides an in-depth look at scientific research into various types of fatty acids, calories, fiber, carbs of foods. Packed with links to scientific studies and complete with an Index. Provides key nutrient data with 26 tables highlighting the components and effects of the foods in our lives. Available in paperback and EBook at Amazon, booksellers, and libraries.

Low Glycemic Happiness 120 Recipes for Blood Sugar Control each recipe provides the Carbohydrate, Glycemic Index (GI), Fiber, Glycemic Load (GL), plus Calories, Fat, Saturated fat, Protein, and Sodium content per serving. Available in paperback and EBook formats at Amazon, booksellers, and libraries.

Are You Sweet Enough Already? Low Glycemic Load desserts For Blood Sugar Control, is available in paperback and EBook formats at Amazon, booksellers, and libraries. These dessert recipes use less common ingredients, like black beans, avocado, and almond flour. These desserts are gluten free, lactose free, and free from table sugar. You will also see the amount of Carbohydrate, Glycemic Index (GI), Fiber, Glycemic Load (GL), Calories, Fat, Saturated fat, Protein, and Sodium content per serving.

Printed in Great Britain
by Amazon